INTERNATIONAL PERSPECTIVES IN PHYSICAL THERAPY 2

Stroke

SERIES EDITORS

Ida Bromley MBE MCSP
Ida Bromley is District Superintendent Physiotherapist at The Royal Free Hospital,
London. A Superintendent Physiotherapist for the past 20 years in hospitals in
England, she has lectured and run workshops in various parts of the U.K., U.S.A.
and South Africa, and written articles for many journals on subjects ranging from
'Rehabilitation of the Severely Disabled' to 'Problem Orientated Medical
Recording'. She is also author of a well-known textbook, *Tetraplegia and Paraplegia*.
From 1978–82, she was Chairman of the Council of the Chartered Society of
Physiotherapy and is currently President of the Organisation of District
Physiotherapists and Vice-President of the Society for Research in Rehabilitation.

Nancy Theilgaard Watts RPT PhD
Nancy Watts is Professor and Director of the Physical Therapy Graduate Program
in the MGH Institute of Health Professions at Massachusetts General Hospital in
Boston. A physical therapy teacher for over 30 years, since 1965 most of her work
has been in establishing advanced study programs for experienced therapists. Her
major academic interests and publications concern methods of clinical teaching,
economics of health care, and analysis of the process of judgment used by clinicians.
Her clinical research has varied widely, ranging from studies of the effects of cold on
spasticity to cost-effectiveness comparisons of different methods of treatment for
common orthopaedic disorders. Dr Watts has served on a number of national and
international commissions, and frequently teaches and consults in Britain,
Scandinavia, and Latin America. She has also helped to prepare physical therapy
teachers for schools in over 20 different countries.

INTERNATIONAL PERSPECTIVES IN PHYSICAL THERAPY 2

Stroke

EDITED BY

Moira A. Banks BA MCSP
Lecturer, Department of Physiotherapy,
The Queen's College, Glasgow

CHURCHILL LIVINGSTONE
EDINBURGH LONDON MELBOURNE AND NEW YORK 1986

CHURCHILL LIVINGSTONE
Medical Division of Longman Group Limited

Distributed in the United States of America by
Churchill Livingstone Inc., 1560 Broadway, New York,
N.Y. 10036, and by associated companies, branches and
representatives throughout the world.

First published 1986

ISBN 0-443-02923-7

ISSN 0267-0380

British Library Cataloguing in Publication Data
Stroke.—(International perspectives in
  physical therapy, ISSN 0267-0380; 2)
  1. Hemiplegia   2. Physical therapy
  I. Banks, Moira A.   II. Series
  616.8'37062   RC385

Library of Congress Cataloging in Publication Data
Main entry under title:
Stroke.
  (International perspectives in physical therapy; 2)
  Bibliography; p.
  Includes index.
  1. Hemiplegics—Rehabilitation.   2. Cerebrovascular
disease—Complications and sequelae—Treatment.
3. Physical therapy.   I. Banks, Moira A.   II. Series.
[DNLM: 1. Cerebrovascular Disorders—rehabilitation.
2. Cerebrovascular Disorders—therapy.   3. Physical
Therapy.   W1 IN827JM v.2 / WL 355 S9189]
RC406.H45S77   1986   616.8'1   85-16589

Produced by Longman Singapore Publishers (Pte) Ltd.
Printed in Singapore

About the Series

The purpose of this series of books is to provide an international exchange of ideas and to explore different approaches in professional therapy practice.

The books will be written primarily for experienced clinicians. They are not intended as basic texts nor as reports on the most recent research, though elements of these aspects may be included.

Articles written by experts from a number of different countries will form the core of each volume. These will be supported by a commentary on the current 'state of the art' in the particular area of practice and an annotated bibliography of key references.

Each volume will cover a topic which we believe to be of universal interest. Some will be concerned with a troublesome symptom, as in this volume; others will be related to problems within a broad diagnostic category, for example sports injuries. Aspects of the organisation of practice and issues of professional concern will be the subjects of future books in the series.

In this volume we have adopted the convention of using 'he' for patient and 'she' for physiotherapist.

We hope that readers will let us have their reactions to the content and format of these publications. Suggestions of other topics considered to be of international interest, which might provide the foci of future volumes would also be welcomed.

I.B
N.T.W

Preface

Hemiplegia from cerebrovascular accident has been a significant cause of impairment and disability in society throughout the ages. The search for methods of alleviating the resulting loss of function and restoring the patient to independence has been the concern of all involved in medicine. However, in the last few decades the major involvement in the treatment of hemiplegia has devolved to the physiotherapist.

Hemiplegia is a catastrophic incident often occurring in a physically and mentally active person, and transforming this individual at a 'stroke' into an emotionally labile, non-communicating, immobile person. This disaster, agonising and isolating as it is for the patient, has far reaching effects on family and friends who find it almost impossible to relate to this unknown and apparently unknowing person. The symptoms of a stroke vary enormously and it is probably in the recognition of the different problems which may occur that most progress has been made. To identify a problem is not necessarily to solve it or to identify methods of alleviating it. Current therapeutic practices, however, have evolved from those which sought to treat isolated symptoms such as spasticity by massage, or loss of movement by local stimulation, to ones which attempt to trigger potential recovery by treating the patient globally. Physiotherapists throughout the world, daily confronted by problems in relation to the rehabilitation of hemiplegia, are looking for help in understanding these problems and in developing relevant programmes of care.

The economic implications of stroke as they relate to health care programmes and to the families of the patients involved, are also of international concern. The timing, duration and method of physiotherapeutic intervention are subjects of discussion and experimentation world-wide, but little concrete information is available.

This volume seeks to promote discussion and exchange of ideas in relation to treatment of hemiplegia by both describing differing approaches to treatment and discussing overall therapeutic management. It is divided into two parts. The first is primarily composed of original papers from physiotherapists working in many parts of the world. Each offers new ideas on the treatment of hemiplegia and identifies areas for further research. The breadth of subjects covered within this section reflects current recognition of the complex nature of problems posed by brain damage. Nevertheless the degree to which certain issues pervade the entire book also reflects current concerns. The second part consists of an annotated bibliography which will enable physiotherapists to become more aware of the breadth of current relevant literature, and to further their own study and research.

Glasgow, 1986   M.B.

Contributors

Moira A. Banks BA MCSP
Lecturer, Department of Physiotherapy, The Queen's College, Glasgow, U.K.

Janet H. Carr DipPhty MA (Columbia) FACP
Senior Lecturer, School of Physiotherapy, Cumberland College of Health Sciences, Lidcombe, N.S.W., Australia

Barbara F.G. Goff ONC MCSP DipTP
Formerly Senior Teacher of Physiotherapy, North Staffs, and Oswestry School of Physiotherapy, U.K.

Caroline Gowland PT MHSc MCPA
Assistant Professor, Department of Neurosciences, McMaster University. Physical therapist (Clinical Specialist in Neurology) at Chedoke – McMaster Hospitals, Hamilton, Ontario, Canada

Iris M. Musa MPhil MCSP DipTP
Teacher, School of Physiotherapy, University Hospital of Wales, Cardiff, U.K.

Roberta B. Shepherd DipPhty MA (Columbia) FACP
Senior Lecturer, School of Physiotherapy, Cumberland College of Health Sciences, Lidcombe, N.S.W., Australia

Maureen Skelly MSc MCSP DipTP
Senior Lecturer in Physiotherapy, University of Ulster, Coleraine, Northern Ireland, U.K.

George Turnbull MCSP DipTP BPT (Manitoba)
Assistant Professor, School of Physiotherapy, Dalhousie University, Halifax, Nova Scotia, Canada

Lotta Widén Holmqvist RPT
Lecturer, Institution of Physical Therapy, Karolinska Institute, Stockholm. Physical Therapist, Huddinge University Hospital, Huddinge, Sweden

Nina Wrethagen RPT
Physical Therapist, Erstagardskiniken, Hasthagsvagen, Nacka, Sweden

Contents

Introduction

The incidence of hemiplegia resulting from cerebrovascular disease has been consistently recorded at around 1.8–2.0 per 1000 population from studies throughout the world (W.H.O., 1971). (Royal College of Physicians of London, 1974). Recently, this figure has been revised following reports noting a declining incidence of cerebrovascular accidents. In a study from the United States, Wenfield (1981) noted a 15% drop between the years 1971 and 1975. Whether this change is related to the success of health education programmes or to greater awareness and more effective control of hypertension is uncertain, but similar trends have been noted elsewhere, and studies in Australia (Barker and Rose, 1984) and the United Kingdom (Acheson and Williams, 1983) indicate that this decline is world wide. However, this trend is unlikely to affect the immediate and obvious need for increasing rehabilitation services.

For those who sustain a cerebrovascular accident the immediate mortality rate is high. Marquardson (1976) in a Danish study reported a 48% mortality rate three weeks after cerebrovascular accident, a figure comparable to a similar British study (Beresford and Weddell, 1979). Weinfield (1981) reviewing survival figures at six months noted a 35% mortality rate in those under seventy five years and 48% in those between seventy-five and eighty-five years.

The increasing incidence of cerebrovascular accidents with advancing years is well documented (Royal College of Physicians of London, 1974; Marquardson, 1976). Generally, in the age group 55–64 the incidence rate is three times greater than in the 45–54 group. For those aged 75–85 this figure increases ten-fold. However, since the immediate mortality is high this increase in incidence though significant is less dramatic. In terms of prevalence, survival after the initial period is closely related to that in the normal population.

When considering the prevalence of cerebrovascular disease in a population it is essential to recognise the significance of the increase in numbers in the 74–85 age group. It has been estimated that in the United Kingdom by the year 2000 there will be an increase in this age group of 33% in the male population and 26% in the female on 1975 figures (Office of Population Census and Surveys, 1980), This implies increasing pressure on current rehabilitation services and indicates a continuing demand for the development of more effective treatment methods and more efficient patterns of delivery of care.

Adams (1974) proposed that improvement in rehabilitation of stroke patients required imaginative and constructive treatment of disordered postural fixation, sensory loss and perceptual barriers. The considerable progress which has been made in the treatment of hemiplegic patients in the last decade may be attributed to an increased awareness by physiotherapists of the importance of sensory and perceptual deficits and their effect on motor learning. However, there is an urgent need for exploration of such subjective views.

The problems which beset objective study of the treatment of stroke are those common to all clinical trials. The variables which potentially may affect outcome are almost unlimited. Some of these variables may be quantifiable but large areas exist in which objective measurements are not possible, for example, the patient's previous mental status and motivation, the degree of family support, and ethnic and social pressures. In addition, the quality of the physical therapy is extremely difficult to measure. Consequently, published studies tend to follow the medical model and, insofar as treatment is concerned, to measure quantity rather than quality of rehabilitation (Wade et al, 1984). Published results focusing on outcome related to gross measurements of function have little influence on the methods and quality of physiotherapy treatment, nor are they necessarily measures of the potential for recovery. The use of other research strategies may permit more effective investigation of more relevant issues including treatment techniques.

Therapeutic development depends upon existing theoretical concepts. Concepts of recovery as they relate to damage to the central nervous system are central to the development of new methods of rehabilitation planning. The concept of irreversible damage in the central nervous system led logically to treatment programmes which emphasised compensatory training of the affected side. The major involvement in the treatment of lower motor neurone disease had conditioned the physical therapist to programmes in which development of muscle strength was paramount where apparent weakness was observed (Voss, 1967). Treatment of upper motor neuron disorders therefore followed this pattern.

The neurodevelopmental concept proposed by Bobath (1970) injected new impetus into the habilitation of the brain-injured child, and later to the rehabilitation of the adult hemiplegic. This concept, which was developed in isolation from concurrent work on the potential plasticity of the central nervous system, led not only to the development of a new therapeutic approach, but was instrumental in stimulating physiotherapists to look to other disciplines for help in relation to motor learning, motivation and restoration of function.

The research findings of neurophysiologists, neuropsychologists, and others from related disciplines, developing the concept of plasticity, the dynamic responses of the central nervous system to injury, have provided the recent basis for current therapy and an incentive for the development of new therapeutic initiatives. This recognition of the therapeutic implications of the results from research laboratories has been a reciprocal process with results being applied in the clinical field and those engaged in the research becoming more aware of its practical application (Moore, 1980; Ince, 1980).

The concept of transferring laboratory results, often gained from animal studies, to clinical practice is scientifically well established. However, effective application requires understanding of all factors which differentiate animal from human studies, particularly those related to behavioural responses. For example, desired behaviour in animal studies may be triggered by noxious stimuli, but this is generally ethically unacceptable in clinical practice and alternative methods of shaping behaviour by, for example reward for achievement, are more likely to be employed.

The clinical application of Taub's (1980) concept of learned non use which is referred to by several contributors to this book may serve as an example of the need for understanding differentiating factors. Early studies (Moss and Sherrington, 1895) had indicated that loss of function followed simple limb deafferentation in animals. Following on the much neglected work of Munk (1905), Taub and his colleagues investigated motor response to deafferentation when accompanied by rehabilitation techniques based on principles of behavioural psychology. They demonstrated that it was possible to restore full function in the deafferented limb provided conditions which demanded and encouraged the use of the affected limb were present. Without these conditions the animal acquired patterns of activity which denied the functional possibilities of the limb—in effect, learned non-used.

Several hypotheses have been developed in order to explain this concept. One such is Taub's inter-limb inhibition hypotheses. This proposed that movement of one fore-limb has an inhibitory effect on movement of the contra-lateral limb. This interlimb mechanism normally held in check by ipsilateral input, is released when such input is removed as in the case of deafferentation. Co-ordinated movement in a symmetrical or reciprocal manner is thus prevented.

This hypothesis may have clinical application. De Souza (1983) described the recovery of a patient who some three weeks after the onset of hemiplegia involving his dominant hand, fell and sustained a Colles fracture of his unaffected wrist. The ensuing functional loss led to an increased need for attempted use of the dominant hemiplegic hand—a condition comparable to that of Taub's animal studies. Good functional recovery followed and the patient ultimately regained fine motor skills including the ability to write. At first he found any action with his affected arm frustrating and acknowledged that had he had function in his non-hemiplegic limb he would not have persisted in attempting movement. Functional need provided the essential stimulus and achievement the reward.

Clinical accounts such as this which include well-documented anecdotal evidence offer valuable therapeutic insights. They help to bridge the gap between laboratory investigation and clinical practice by identifying factors necessary for successful therapeutic application. Brodal, a Norwegian neuro-anatomist, carefully recorded (1973) his recovery from a left-sided hemiplegia. Several interesting points emerge from his description but notable features are his persistence in attempting self re-education and his involvement in the processes of rehabilitation. Bach-y-Rita (1980) recorded the recovery of function in a patient with hemiplegia of his dominant side following brain stem infarction. The author noted that the patient was extremely active in his own rehabilitation and was willing to work hard over a period of years. One example of this motivation was that, although able to write with his unaffected hand, he refused to do so, preferring to embark on the task of learning to type using his affected hand. At first this skill was slow and accompanied by many errors but over the ensuing months increase in speed and accuracy was achieved. Some three years later the patient returned to full employment. A significant feature of both accounts was the high level of self-motivation.

The importance of motivation in successful rehabilitation has never been questioned. Its significance in the treatment of the brain injured is arguably even greater. Brodal (1976) has proposed that in some mystical way motivation may be directly involved in the physiological processes of recovery by influencing sprouting in the remaining nerve cells. Despite such intriguing speculation, the role of motivation in the treatment of hemiplegic patients remains poorly investigated. Finger and Stein (1982), while regretting the absence of controlled studies in this field, suggest that motivation may be one of the most important factors in rehabilitation where the ultimate goal is recovery of function. The observation by Belmont et al (1969) that patients with brain damage are less well motivated to work on their own than others with comparable neurological lesions, makes the need for investigation the more urgent. Moore (1980) proposed that one important goal of the therapeutic team concerned with recovery of function must be the motivation of the patient until such time as self-motivation is established.

In the early stages, motivation will have been initiated and fostered by the enthusiasm and energy of the therapeutic team. Motivation is most likely to continue if clear recognition and approval accompany the patient's early endeavours and achievements. The active involvement of all concerned with the patient's welfare, including relatives and friends, in developing and determining a rehabilitation strategy is essential if confusion and frustration are not to erode initial motivation.

The transition from an externally motivated programme to one which is self-motivated and self-perpetuating is largely dependent on the degree to which the patient can be helped to understand the philosophy of the rehabilitation programme. This will require his involvement in discussion concerning treatment principles and his acceptance of the demands which these will make upon him. In stressing the need to educate and involve patients in their own therapy, Weed (1973) suggested that patients may represent the greatest paramedical force in the health service. Treatment programmes are most likely to be self-motivating where they directly acknowledge the patient's perceived needs. The tendency of programmes to reflect the aspirations of the therapist rather than those of the patient may well be reflected in loss of motivation. This discrepancy between the therapists' objectives and the patients' perceived need has been explored by Partridge (1984). She calls for much more discussion between therapist and patient in establishing both short-term and long-term goals which are mutually acceptable, meaningful and achievable.

Maintenance of the momentum of rehabilitation in the later and less dramatic period of recovery raises different issues for therapist and patient. Continued motivation in both patient and all concerned with his welfare is difficult to maintain. Conflicting beliefs concerning the possibility of further recovery and economic pressures which tend towards withdrawal of support are significant in determining further therapeutic strategies. Studies reporting little recovery after six months (Brocklehurst et al, 1978; Stern et al, 1970; Licht, 1975) conclude that physiotherapy beyond six months after the onset of hemiplegia is both economically wasteful and therapeutically ineffective. This view contrasts markedly with other accounts of therapeutic outcome following brain damage (Levine, 1952; Brodal, 1973; Bach-y-Rita, 1980) which note continuing recovery over much longer periods.

The effects of these conflicting studies on those directly involved with the patient's rehabilitation must be considered when assessing long-term motivation. The influence of expectations on outcome is well known. Strupp and Luvborsky (1962) confirmed the relationship between expectations by therapists of outcome and actual outcome of care. Therefore, predictions that little recovery will take place after six months are likely to have an adverse influence on further progress.

When the end of the six-month period coincides with discharge from formal rehabilitation, which may often be the case, this action may well be interpreted by the patient as signalling the end of hope for further recovery, and by the therapist as further disillusionment in relation to her specific skills. For the patient at this time there may be the onset of depression (Langton Hewer, 1976) or of what Robinson (1976) refers to 'as a period of unhappiness and quiet dispair'. The future seems bleak and despite exhortations to continue exercising the motivation to do so is absent. The concept of success is lost and effort no longer produces satisfaction. For the therapist there is confirmation of negative predicitons.

Feigenson (1981) reviewing alternative patterns of care noted the lack of information on outcomes and cost. Some studies have been done which compare one pattern of care with another. Garraway et al (1980) comparing the outcome of therapy carried out in a stroke unit with that in a traditional medical unit reported an increase in the proportion of patients classified as independent at the time of discharge from the stroke unit. This improvement was not, however, sustained when patients were interviewed one year later. The effect of variation in intensity of physiotherapy following discharge from hospital has been investigated by Smith et al (1981). Those receiving intensive therapy showed greatest improvement. When reviewed one year later the group who had received no formal rehabilitation but were regularly visited by a health visitor and encouraged to continue exercising showed a significant deterioration when assessed on an activities-of-daily-living scale compared to those who had intensive physiotherapy. Results of studies such as these indicate the need for investigation of alternative patterns of care together with the characteristics of patients for whom they are best suited.

Physiotherapists involved in the rehabilitation of patients following cerebrovascular accidents face two distinct tasks. Firstly, they must continue to develop more effective means of treating the immediate disorder. This requires refinement of existing techniques and the introduction and development of new techniques based on the results of research in a variety of disciplines. In addition there is a need for innovation and experimentation in the delivery of treatment in hospitals and in the community. The effects of varied intensity and frequency of treatment during what is now believed to be a critical period in the reorganisation of brain function remains obscure, but they must be identified if patients are to be enabled to develop their full functional potential. Secondly, strategies designed to maintain and develop motivation in the long term must be explored. Lane (1978) identified the need to teach therapeutic skills to those who support and care for the patient. This long-term approach to rehabilitation requires considerable changes in attitude from all concerned with the patient's immediate treatment. It also requires change from those less intimately involved in the patient's care but influential in his management. Effective use of voluntary and unskilled assistance in maintaining motivation and interest in the patient and in his immediate supporters must be explored. The innovative use of modern technology as a stimulus to learning may be one way in which the patient may maintain performance in the absence of the therapist. Active collaboration by therapists in the development and use of modern technology as a rehabilitation tool for the treatment of hemiplegia must be pursued.

The contributors to this book have responded to the need for continuing evolution of treatment techniques and rehabilitation strategies for hemiplegia. Each chapter records individual developments but throughout the book several issues emerge as being of general concern.

Firstly, there is considerable recognition of the degree to which hemiplegia is a family illness. The disruptive effect of impairment will be felt not only by the patient but by those who surround him. The effect on therapeutic outcome of those surrounding the patient is being increasingly acknowledged (Mulhall, 1981; Kinsella, 1980).

Several contributors to this book refer to this whether by noting, as Gowland does, that the degree of family support available is one predictor of outcome, or, as Carr and Shepherd, Goff and Widen Holmqvist and Wrethagen do, by advocating active involvement of relatives and friends in the rehabilitation process.

A second issue of general concern is the nature of the environment in which rehabilitation takes place. Widen Holmqvist and Wrethagen stress the importance of ensuring that those who care for and support the patient are knowledgeable about treatment principles and methods, and skilful in their implementation. Several authors draw attention to the need for positive attitudes by all caring for the patients concerning ultimate outcome. Turnbull discusses the way in which maximum physical environmental stimulation may occur on the affected side, and Carr and Shepherd stress the need for patterns of activity which as nearly as possible simulate a normal day's routine. In considering this aspect, it is salutary to compare the enriched environment in which the brain damaged child is habilitated with the deprived situation in which the adult hemiplegic is rehabilitated.

The importance of sensation in re-educating function is acknowledged by many contributors to this book. Each author has a different emphasis, but its importance in the initiation and control of movement is fully recognised. Skelly advocates substitution and augmentation of disordered or absent sensory feedback in re-educating movement. Goff emphasises the importance of afferent input in achieving motor control. Turnbull stresses the need for sensory feedback on both the quality of the performed skill and its resulting action. Motor problems arising from cerebrovascular accidents are well recognised but the role of disordered sensation in perpetuating these problems is not fully understood. Much work still needs to be done on the integration of sensory and motor re-education programmes.

Prediction of outcome following stroke is of considerable concern to both patient and therapist. For the patient and his family it is of immediate concern for future planning of their life-style. For the therapist the importance of predicting outcome has a different significance. Resources for the treatment of hemiplegia are finite and it is important that they are used to maximum effectiveness. The question of whom will benefit most from the use of such services must be of concern to all planning rehabilitation services. Prediction of outcome following hemiplegia is notoriously difficult since 'the tendency to improvement is very marked and makes it difficult to estimate the actual influence of treatment.' (Gowers, 1893). Currently, most predictions made are subjective and arise from the therapists' intuitive use of cumulated experience. Gowland, in her chapter on outcome following stroke, describes an objective method of predicting recovery levels following hemiplegia. The potential use of such a measure is exciting. It offers the possibility of determining priorities in a rational manner and of allocating resources accordingly. Since a predicted base line of outcome may be established, variation in treatment methods and modes may be evaluated.

Gowland's chapter will undoubtedly raise many questions. One may well relate to the degree to which those treating patients react to prediction of outcome. It may be anticipated that some physiotherapists will respond in a self-fulfilling way and the outcome of their therapy then will reflect that which was predicted. For others, predictions of outcome may provide an incentive to develop programmes which aim to achieve higher functional levels.

Recovery of independent gait is for many hemiplegics an important goal in any rehabilitation programme. Musa discusses gait re-education from the perspective of physiological studies. Many physiotherapists have reservations about therapeutic principles which are derived from studies on lower animals, but from such studies Musa logically and convincingly traces the essential elements of gait control and confirms their importance in man. She identifies certain factors which are essential for re-education of normal gait patterns and in doing so indicates a method of measuring quality and quantity of gait. Her findings confirm the empirical observation of many practitioners, and identify essential aspects of gait re-education. They will also provide a stimulus for those concerned with qualitative aspects of therapy.

The chapter by Carr and Shepherd on motor training contains examples of a therapeutic approach which has evolved from careful evaluation of laboratory studies. The findings of many disciplines have been culled in developing their approach to motor training and this methodology may provide a useful model for others. This chapter not only reports and discusses the results of these studies and their practical therapeutic implications, but also identifies issues which may have even more general therapeutic application. For example, the need for accurate evaluation of the patient's problem is an essential part of the motor training programme. The patient's movement patterns are analysed so that missing components may be identified. A therapeutic hypothesis is formed and treatment methods chosen. Without this evaluation of outcome it is impossible. This philosophy is appropriate not only for treatment of brain damaged patients but also for other patient groups.

The authors' approach to treating elderly and hemiplegic patients is both reasoned and positive. Many whose work extends to other specialist areas may find such an approach equally relevant.

Pain in the shoulder joint following hemiplegia is common; it is distressing for the patient and often provides a serious obstacle for rehabilitation. This chapter includes a section which discusses possible causes of this problem and methods of management.

Some statements made by the authors may be thought provoking, for example their view on the development of spasticity may be at variance with other's experience. It is interesting to compare their expectation of recovery of hand function with that of other contributors to this book.

Two chapters in this book are particularly concerned with the role of sensation in motor re-education. Goff explores and expands the therapeutic concepts originally described by Rood and relates these to more recent neurophysiological findings. Skelly is concerned to augment deficient sensory feedback or to substitute one sensory modality for another in retraining movement.

The diverse nature of brain damage following a cerebrovascular accident may make the initiation of a motor response difficult in the early stages of re-education. In patients who are unable to co-operate because of confusion or receptive loss this difficulty may persist. Methods described by Goff enable motor responses to occur in the absence of conscious co-operation from the patient, and enable treatment to begin at an early stage. The lack of neurophysiological evidence in support of these techniques has, in the past, led to an aura of mysticism surrounding their use. Recent neurophysiological studies have gone some way towards altering this state although much remains unexplained. Therapeutic techniques, however, have often been used successfully in advance of physiological understanding which has followed later.

Goff's approach to treatment of hemiplegia uses treatment principles which are at variance with those of other contributors to this book. Such conflict is inevitable in an evolving practice. An appendix has been included which will enable the physiotherapist to become familiar with the use of these techniques, thus enabling evaluation and development of their most appropriate application.

The relationship between sensation and movement is further explored by Skelly. Interesting issues are raised related to the control of normal movement and the effect of disruption on complex systems. The review of the research literature identifies some of these questions and the section on modes of biofeedback action offers new thinking on possible explanations. In discussing these, Skelly recognises the need for further study and research in this area. This chapter not only encourages clinical research into the use of biofeedback but makes it possible for physiotherapists to undertake it.

Techniques such as those described by Goff and Skelly are essentially therapeutic tools for facilitating specific motor responses in patients. It is important to recognise that for maximum effectiveness they must not be used in isolation but within a total rehabilitation programme.

Turnbull approaches retraining of the hemiplegic from a different perspective. He calls for understanding of motor skill acquisition processes for effective use of any chosen treatment method. Many of the problems excounted in motor re-education may be more easily understood in this framework. His study has widespread implications and requires physiotherapists to identify those aspect of a patient's performance which reflect incomplete learning when planning treatment programmes. The alternative methods of delivery of care he proposes may prompt others to further such innovation.

Consistent methods of facilitating movement and opportunity for practising newly regained motor skills have been recognised by many as important for successful rehabilitation following brain damage. This is more likely to be achieved when those involved in the patient's immediate care are aware of both the treatment principles being followed and their practical application. This requires carefully planned interaction and Widen Holmqvist and Wrethagen describe educational programmes to meet such needs. These programmes have been carefully constructed to ensure that the patient's problems are recognised and their needs met.

Significant use is made of role-play as a teaching method in addition to the use of more traditional methods. The value of simulation in creating awareness of problems posed by physical disability has in some areas been recognised. Its use in enabling those caring for the hemiplegic patient to appreciate the resulting physical limitations is less common. For example, personal experience of being fed or of attempting to swallow while in an abnormal postural position, may be particularly valuable in developing awareness of the factors necessary for good therapeutic practice.

The authors of this chapter also recognise that many are involved in total care and that it must extend over 24 hours. All levels and grades of staff, including night staff, are therefore involved in these programmes.

The importance of family support on rehabilitation outcomes is also clearly demonstrated in this chapter. Formally constructed group sessions may not be immediately achievable in every rehabilitation situation but the value to all of consultation and discussion between members of the therapeutic team and the patient's relatives is clearly demonstrated by Widen Holmqvist and Wrethagen. Use of formal evaluation techniques has been an important factor in their development and must be an integral part of such educational programmes.

It is the purpose of this book to promote discussion and further study and research in the treatment of hemiplegia. Each author has contributed to this aim by exploring areas requiring further work and by identifying unanswered questions. Those reading this book may find apparent conflict in the basic underlying philosophies proposed, but it is only by exploring these issues and furthering the research basis of physiotherapy that progress may be made.

REFERENCES

Acheson R M, Williams D R R 1983 Does consumption of fruit and vegetables protect against stroke? Lancet: 1191–1193
Adams G F 1974 Cerebrovascular disability and the ageing brain. Churchill Livingstone, Edinburgh
Bach-y-rita P 1980 Brain plasticity as a basis for therapeutic procedures. In: Bach-y-Rita P (ed) Recovery of function: theoretical considerations for brain injury rehabilitation. Hans Huber Publishers, Bern
Barker D J P, Rose G 1984 Epidemiology in medical practice, Churchill Livingstone, Edinburgh
Belmont I, Benjamin H, Ambrose J, Restuccia R D 1969 Effect of cerebral damage on motivation in rehabilitation. Archives of Physical Medicine and Rehabilitation 9:507
Beresford S A A, Weddell J M 1979 Planning for stroke patients. HMSO, London

Bobath B 1970 Adult hemiplegia evaluation and treatment, Heinemann Medical Books Ltd, London

Brocklehurst J C, Andrews K, Morris P E, Richards B, Laycock P J 1978 Medical, social and psychological aspects of stroke, University of Manchester, England

Brodal A 1973 Self-observation and neuro-anatomical consideration after a stroke. Brain 96: 675–694

Brodal A 1976 Personal communication, quoted in: Bach-y-Rita, P (ed) Recovery of function: theoretical considerations for brain injury rehabilitation. Hans Huber Publishers, Bern

De Souza L H 1983 The effects of sensation and motivation on regaining movement control following stroke, Physiotherapy 69(7): 238–240

Feigenson J S 1981 Stroke rehabilitation: outcome studies and guidelines for alternative levels of care. Stroke 1(3): 372–375

Finger S, Stein D G 1982 Brain damage and recovery, Academic Press, New York

Garraway W M et al 1979 The declining incidence of stroke. The New England Journal of Medicine, 300(9): 449–452

Gowers W R 1893 A manual of diseases of the nervous system. J & A Churchill, London, Vol II, p 447

Ince L P 1980 Behavioural psychology in rehabilitation medicine: clinical applications. Williams & Wilkins, Baltimore

Kinsella G J, Duffy F D 1980 Attitudes towards disability expressed by spouses of stroke patients. Scandanavian Journal of Rehabilitation 12 (Pt II): 73–76

Lane R E J 1978 Facilitation of weight transference in the stroke patient. Physiotherapy 64(9):260–264

Langton H R 1976 Stroke rehabilitation In: Gillingham F J, Mawdsley C, Williams A E (eds) Stroke. Churchill Livingstone, Edinburgh

Levine J 1952 Relative effects of occipital and peripheral blindness upon intellectual Functions. Archives of Neurology and Psychiatry 67: 310–314

Licht S (ed) 1965 Therapeutic exercise. Waverley Press, Baltimore, pp 426–468

Licht S 1975 Stroke and its rehabilitation. Waverly press, Baltimore

Marquardson J 1975 Follow-up of stroke patients. Age & Ageing, Supplement: 41–48

Moore J 1980 Neuro-anatomical considerations relating to recovery of function following brain injury. In: Bach-y-Rita P (ed) Recovery of function: theoretical considerations for brain injury rehabilitation. Hans Huber Publishers, Bern

Mott F W, Sherrington C S 1895 Experiments upon the influence of sensory nerves upon movement and nutrition of the limbs. Proceedings of the Royal Society 57: 481–488

Munk H 1909 Ueber Die Functionen von Hirn und Ruckenmark. Hirshwald, Berlin, pp 247–285

Mulhall D J 1981 Stroke: A problem for patient and family. Physiotherapy 67(7): 195–197

Office of Census and Surveys 1980 Population projections 1978–2018. HMSO London

Partridge C J 1984 Recovery from conditions involving physical disability. Physiotherapy 70(6): 233–236

Robinson R A 1976 Psychiatric aspects of stroke. In: Gillingham F J, Mawdsley C, Williams A E (eds) Stroke. Churchill Livingstone, Edinburgh

Royal College of Physicians of London 1974 Report of the geriatrics committee working group on strokes.

Smith D S et al 1981 Remedial therapy after stroke: a randomised controlled trial. British Medical Journal 282: 517–524

Stern P H, McDowel F, Miller J M, Robinson M 1970 Factors influencing stroke rehabilitation. Stroke 2: 231–215

Stern P H, McDowell F, Miller J M, Robinson M 1970 Effects of facilitation exercise techniques in stroke rehabilitation. Archives of Physical Medicine and Rehabilitation 51: 526–531

Taub E 1980 Somatosensory deafferentation research with monkeys: implication for rehabilitation medicine. In: Ince L P (ed)Behavioural psychology in rehabilitation medicine: Clinical applications. Williams & Wilkins, Baltimore

Voss D E 1967 Proprioceptive Neuromuscular Facilitation. American Journal of Physical Medicine 46(1)

Wade D T, Skilbeck, C E, Langton Hewer, R L, Wood V A 1984 Therapy after stroke—determinants and effects, Int Rehabit Med: 6: 105–110

Weed L L 1973 Problem oriented records: can it work in general practice? Medical Recording Service Foundation, Audio Tape 73/10, Royal College of General Practitioners

Weinfield F D (ed) 1981 The national survey of stroke. Supplement No 1, Stroke, Vol 12, No 2. The American Heart Association Inc, Dallas

World Health Organization 1971 Technical report series. Cerebro-vascular disease, prevention, treatment & rehabilitation, W.H.O., Geneva

Predicting the outcome of stroke

The knowledge gained from accurately predicting various aspects of post-stroke recovery could be applied to the design of more effective and efficient treatment programmes. For example, the ability to judge which stroke survivors might be expected to regain functional recovery of the hemiplegic arm could determine the choice of a physical therapy programme appropriate to the expected outcome.

The decision to provide an intensive in-patient rehabilitation programme for a stroke patient should be based on the prospect of individual patients benefiting from such a programme—the benefits being measured in terms of improved survival rate, more favourable discharge disposition, reduced length of hospital stay and/or improved functional outcomes. Costly programmes with little or no rehabilitative effect are recognized as poor rehabilitative practice.

Although the stroke literature contains documentation of the anticipated outcomes and clinical findings of prognostic significance that can help members of the health care team assess a patient's rehabilitative potential, there is a paucity of scientific evidence regarding the expected changes in those aspects of the patient's physical status that are commonly the physical therapist's concern. Moreover, specific predictive equations for accurately estimating these expected changes are not available. When therapists are asked to provide a prediction, it is generally based on intuition.

This chapter's purpose is to address this issue by providing physical therapists with information that can be used in the prediction of post-rehabilitation sensori-motor recovery. For presentation purposes, this information is divided into two sections. The first section provides a review of the existing body of knowledge, while the second section adds to this knowledge by reporting on a study that analyzes information on those specific aspects of physical status that are commonly the physical therapist's concern. In both sections the subject is discussed under the headings recovery magnitude, prognostic indicators and predictions. The second section, that describing the study, has a fourth component, a prospective study, aimed at evaluating the predictive validity of equations identified.

A review of the literature demonstrates that the magnitude of physical recovery, prognostic indicators and predictions as they pertain to certain aspects of post-stroke outcome have already received some attention. Therefore, before reporting on the particular predictive aspects examined by the study, we will examine the relevant information available.

THE LITERATURE REVIEW

Ellinson (1974) states that outcomes, or the end results of health satisfaction, contain measures of death/life, disease/health, disability/activity, discomfort/ease, and dissatisfaction/satisfaction. The specific outcomes found in the stroke rehabilitation literature that refer to the above list include: (1) survival, (2) discharge disposition, (3) length of stay, (4) functional status, and (5) neurological status. These outcome measures serve in the evaluation of recovery, in the measurement of the effects of rehabilitation, and in the determination of measures of prognostic significance.

Under functional status (No. 4 above) can be found a discussion of the recovery magnitude of ambulation and hand function—aspects of a patient's physical status commonly assessed by physical therapists and the ones pertinent to this article.

Recovery magnitude

Commenting on the ambulation status of stroke patients following rehabilitation, Waylonis et al (1973) found that 65% of these patients ambulated independently, 7% were ambulating with supervision and 23% were non-ambulatory. Other authors (Moskowitz et al, 1972; Steinberg, 1973; Feigenson et al, 1977) reported that from 61 to 85% regained independent ambulation.

The recovery of function of the upper limb presents a more dismal picture than that of ambulation. Those authors (Adams & McComb, 1953; Joshi et al, 1974) who did comment specifically on the percentage of patients with functional recovery of the upper limb found it to be 4 and 5% respectively. It was noted, however, that physical recovery of the upper limb could take place without return of function; Bard and Hirschberg (1965), for instance, reported that about 40% of their subjects recovered full voluntary

motion of the upper limb. This rate concurs with the findings of
Moscowitz et al (1972) who stated that 37% of the patients they
evaluated had normal to good hand recovery as measured by
strength, lack of contractures and reduced spasticity. These findings indicate that a functional hand is dependent on more than just
voluntary range of movement and strength. Indeed, unless the
stroke survivor is capable of moving his fingers individually, with the
normal timing and coordination required to manipulate objects in
a functional manner, he will not perceive his hand as being functional. This assessment contrasts with that of the leg, which is
considered functional once the patient reambulates, regardless of
the quality of the gait.

The stroke rehabilitation literature makes no mention of balance,
gross motor performance or lower limb mobility as measures of
physical outcome. These, along with upper limb mobility and gait,
could provide valuable information in predicting the potential for
recovery of physical function.

Prognostic indicators

Prognostic indicators are objective clinical features, or patient
characteristics, that aid in the prediction of outcome. Ordinarily
they cannot be used alone to provide a precise prediction; instead
they function as general indicators and are particularly valuable
when used in combination with each other. As observed earlier,
prognostic indicators vis-a-vis stroke patients have been identified
for such various outcomes as survival, discharge disposition, length
of stay, and functional and neurological status, each of which is
outlined below.

Survival

The prognosis for survival has been found to be adversely affected
by hemianopsia, prolonged deep unconsciousness, advanced age,
severe hypertension, bloodstained cerebrospinal fluid, a severe co-
existing disease, or poor functional recovery (Waylonis et al, 1973;
MacLeod & Williamson, 1972).

Discharge disposition

The authors of one paper (Lehmann et al, 1975) found family
income and involvement to be the only feature that correlated with

a favourable discharge disposition. They found no such correlation between disposition and (a) extensive heart lesion, (b) signs of congestive heart failure, (c) generalized arteriosclerosis, (d) gross perceptual deficit, (e) lower education, or (f) advanced age. Feigenson et al (1977) adding to the list of factors affecting discharge disposition, included severity of the weakness, time interval from the onset of the stroke to admission for rehabilitative care, non-ambulation, and dependence on others for bowel and bladder care. Heminsensory loss, however, has no prognostic significance.

Length of stay

Stern et al (1971) and Feigenson et al (1977) both noted that the patients' length of stay in hospital is adversely affected by the severity of involvement and persistent non-ambulation. In addition, hemiparesis in the presence of severe organic mental syndrome, severe perceptual dysfunction or poor motivation reportedly indicates a poor prognosis (Feigenson et al, 1977). Hemisensory loss and side of hemiplegia have no prognostic significance for length of stay (Feigenson et al, 1977; Mills & DiGenio, 1983).

Functional status

Self-care. Several features (previous cerebrovascular disease, bowel and bladder incontinence, low self-care scores at time of admission, elevated systolic blood pressure, and amount of time between the onset of stroke and the start of the rehabilitation program) have been shown to indicate a poor prognosis for self-care (Feigenson et al, 1977). Feigenson et al (1977) reported that the degree of the severity of weakness at time of admission was the strongest predictor of independence in activities of daily living. These investigators also observed that hemiparesis accompanied by organic mental syndrome, perceptual dysfunction or poor motivation resulted in a poor prognosis. Side of hemiplegia has no prognostic significance (Mills & Degenio, 1983).

Ambulation. Moscowitz et al (1972) found that a hemisensory defect adversely affects ambulation status. Feigenson et al (1977), however, found no such relationship and reported that the severity of the weakness at the point of admission to the rehabilitation program and hemiparesis in the presence of other syndromes acted as prognostic indicators of ambulation status.

Rehabilitative potential. Patients found 'less likely to improve on a rehabilitation program' generally include those with an extensive severe lesion, signs of congestive heart failure, generalized arteriosclerosis, gross perceptual deficits, lower education, advanced age, bowel incontinence of three to four weeks duration, left-versus right-sided hemiplegia, and delayed initiation of treatment (Adams & McComb, 1953; Lorenze & Cancro, 1962; Peszczyniski, 1963; Anderson, 1967; Lehmann et al, 1975; Feigenson et al, 1977). Once again heminsensory loss does not correlate with rehabilitative potential (Feigenson et al, 1977).

Neurological status

Stern et al (1971) found that motility (that is, tapping rate and accuracy of placement of the upper and lower extremity) and strength are affected by the severity of the involvement. In that same study, the hemiparetic patient showed a mean improvement that was about twice that of the patient with complete hemiplegia: the passage of time between the occurrence of stroke and the start of the rehabilitation program also adversely affected the prognosis for improved motility (1971).

By using more sensitive statistical techniques such as multivariate regression analysis, one can determine equations to aid in predicting outcome.

Predictions

Three studies in the stroke literature have reported using regression analysis for predicting outcome. The outcome of interest in two of these studies (Anderson et al, 1974; Wade et al, 1983) was ADL, while in the third study, that by Ben-Yishay et al (1970), length of stay and ambulation as well as ADL were investigated.

The first study (Bourestom, 1967; Bourestom & Howard, 1968; Anderson et al, 1974; Gersten, 1975) analyzed the relationship between over 600 independent or predictor variables and improvement in Kenny ADL score at time of discharge from hospital and again at a three month follow-up. Three categories of variables, that is, medical and nursing, behavioral, and demographic and environmental, differentiated among self-care improvement groups at statistically reliable levels. From the list of medical and nursing variables analyzed, ten were found to be significant, with the first four appearing the most frequently in the equations developed

(Anderson et al, 1974). The ten variables were: time since onset, urinary continence, pain and temperature sense, standing balance, fecal continence, strength of hip extensors, decubitus ulcer, tongue protrusion, toe position sense and history of a previous CVA. From the list of behavioral variables, the performance IQ of the WAIS, the Porteus maze test and part B of the trail making test were able to differentiate groups reliably, and from the list of demographic and environmental variables (Bourestom 1967; Bourestom & Howard, 1968), seven variables, that is, education level, age, marital status, occupational rating, source of income, gender and socioeconomic status appeared in the equations developed (Anderson et al, 1974).

Wade et al (1983) analyzed the relationship between data obtained from the initial post-stroke assessment and a patient's actual ADL acore on the Barthel scale at a fixed interval, six months after stroke. The variables identified as providing significant predictive information were urinary incontinence, a motor deficit in the arm, sitting balance, hemianopsia and age. The equation generated accounted for 38% of the total variance in outcome.

Ben-Yishay et al (1970) studied only patients who had suffered left-sided hemiplegia. Forty two predictor variables, thirty six of which came from psychometric tests, were analyzed to determine their ability to provide significant predictive information for outcomes of self care, hospital stay to the nearest month and ambulation status. All three outcomes could be reliably predicted using the complete list of variables analyzed. However, the psychometric testing for each patient took close to three hours to complete, this not including the time required to record the six demographic characteristics identified.

In this present study, the outcomes for which predictive equations were sought were not limited to ADL function and ambulation but were expanded to include several additional aspects of sensori-motor recovery considered to be important in the practice of physical therapy.

THE STUDY

The overall purpose of the study was to identify objective information for reliably predicting sensori-motor recovery post-stroke rehabilitation.

A 'stroke' was defined as a neurological result of an ischaemic brain lesion caused by arteriosclerotic or embolic occlusion or haemorrhage with resulting hemiplegia, hemiparesis or bilateral involvement.

To accomplish the overall objective of predicting sensori-motor recovery, the study was divided into four components. The objectives of these components were:

(i) to describe the magnitude of the physical recovery. This included a description of the recovery that occurred in the hemiplegic arm and leg, gross motor performance and gait;

(ii) to determine the relationship between prognostic indicators and outcome. The relationship between six important patient characteristics (i.e., sensation, perception, severity of the hemiplegia, age, length of time from onset and side of hemiplegia), the prognostic indicators, and the recovery magnitude of the four aspects of physical status, the arm, leg, gross motor performance and gait, was analyzed;

(iii) to provide physical therapists with clinically useful equations for predicting the level of sensori-motor recovery following stroke rehabilitation, while indicating the relative value of commonly assessed patient characteristics. To accomplish this third objective, the relationship was sought between 14 dependent or outcome variables of sensori-motor performance (i.e. length of patient stay, perception, sensation, stage of arm, stage of leg, postural control, gross motor performance, gait, discharge disposition, shoulder pain, locomotion, ADL, gait aides and speed of walk) and a set of 23 independent or criterion variables (i.e., ADL, age, gender, side of hemiplegia, handedness, weeks post-stroke, length of stay, aphasia, perception, sensation, number of complications, stage of arm, stage of leg, postural control, gross motor performance, gait, CTT scan, artery involved, family support, locomotion, urinary continence, mental status and shoulder pain);

(iv) to test the accuracy of the predictive equations developed (in iii above) by conducting a prospective study on a new population sample.

Method

The study was carried out at a rehabilitation centre* where inpatients receive intensive rehabilitation from a multidisciplinary team consisting of a physiatrist, nurse, physical therapist, occupational

* Chedoke Rehabilitation Centre, Chedoke-McMaster Hospitals, Hamilton, Ontario.

therapist, speech therapist, social worker, orthotist and neuropsychologist. The patients studied received physical therapy daily, Monday to Friday. The physical therapy emphasized a 'hands-on' neuro-faciliatory approach incorporating commonly accepted principles of facilitation and inhibition. A complete description of the therapy including the rationale, description, goals and mechanics is contained in an internal report (Torresin et al, 1982)* of the Centre.

Characteristics of the population

In total, a population of 335 patients admitted between 1973 and 1982 were included in the study. However, study components one and two were completed in 1978 and included only 223 patients. These patients were consecutive admissions from 1973 to 1977. Components three and four included data coming from the entire population.

A total data base had not been gathered on the first 223 admissions. Information not available on these patients included: mental status; family support; artery involved; CTT scan; Kenny ADL, locomotion and bladder status; postural control; number of gait aides; speed of walk; shoulder pain and discharge disposition. Data on these variables came from the assessment of the 112 subsequent admissions only.

Information on primary diagnosis, gender, side of involvement, time from onset of stroke, length of stay, complicating factors, communicative abilities, perceptual status, stage of recovery of the arm and leg, gait status, gross motor performance and sensation was available from the entire population.

All 335 patients had a primary diagnosis of stroke. 174 were male, 161 female. 175 had right-sided, 172 left-sided and 8 patients bilateral involvement. The median time from the onset of the stroke to admission to the Centre was six weeks, with a range of one week to five years. The median length of stay was seven weeks, ranging from one to 49 weeks.

Complication factors were noted, and it was found that major complications accompanied the stroke in 237 patients, with 152 of these having more than one problem. Included in the list of

---

* *Treatment guidelines for motor recovery in hemiplegic patients: postural control, upper extremities, lower extremities and gait* is available from Chedoke Rehabilitation Centre, M.P.O. Box 2000, Stn. A., Hamilton, Ontario L8N 3Z5

complications were limb amputations, seizures, chronic obstructive lung disease, chronic open wounds, kidney disease, a major surgical procedure during hospital stay, rheumatoid arthritis, an acute fractured hip, schizoprenia, dementia, polio, Parkinson's disease, bilateral peripheral neuropathies, cancer, myocardial and pulmonary infarctions and duodenal ulcers.

The patients were evaluated for a variety of reasons before undergoing the specific physical therapy tests. When an aphasia was evident, the patient's communicative abilities were objectively evaluated by a speech therapist using the Porch index of communicative ability (Porch, 1972). Of 334 patients, 73 had a complete functional loss of communicative ability (global aphasia), 42 had a moderate loss, and 219 had functional speech.

The perceptual status of all patients was evaluated unless the patient's general medical condition, or communicative or mental status, precluded testing. Evaluations were done by an occupational therapist using an objective assessment (OSOT, undated). In total, 276 patients were evaluated. Patients who scored below 50% on the assessment were considered to be perceptually impaired for the purpose of this study. Whereas 111 patients were found to be impaired, 165 were termed only mildly involved or normal.

Information on family support was available for 108 patients; 100 were classified as having a supportive family, 6 no family and 2 no family involved with the rehabilitation process although family had been identified. 102 of 112 patients, were deemed to have involvement in the territory supplied by the middle cerebral artery. CTT scans were available on 25 patients, 6 scans identified haemorrhage and 13 infarction as the cause of the CVA. 6 scans were normal.

Physical therapy tests

Using a set form, a physical therapist assessed each patient at the time of admission to and discharge from the Centre. Aspects rated included the patient's stage of motor recovery of the arm and leg, gait or ambulation status, gait speed, number of gait aids used, postural control, gross motor performance, sensation, severity of paralysis and shoulder pain.

Stage of motor recovery of the arm and leg. The recovery stage of each patient was evaluated according to the Brunnstrom (Brunnstrom, 1970) criteria (Fig. 2.1), a method of assessment that has been standardized by Fugl-Meyer et al (1975). An unstandardized

STAGE	CHARACTERISTICS
Stage 1	No active movement present
Stage 2	Basic limb synergies either appear as weak associated reactions or appear on attempted voluntary movement. Spasticity begins to develop
Stage 3	Basic limb synergies or components of these synergies are performed voluntarily and show definite joint movements. Spasticity is marked.
Stage 4	Movement combinations begin to deviate from basic limb synergies.
Stage 5	There is relative independence from the basic limb synergies and the patient has the ability to mix difficult extensor synergy with flexor synergy movements. Spasticity decreases further.
Stage 6	Isolated joint movements are performed in a well-coordinated manner.

Fig. 2.1 Brunnstrom stages of motor recovery of the arm and leg (from Physiotherapy Canada 34: 77–84, 1982).

but more sensitive adaptation* of the Fugl-Mayer assessment was used in this study. (A four-point instead of a three-point scale was developed so that the previous midpoint of the scale—classified as 'some movement present'—could be subdivided into two sections, that is 'movement less than half range' and 'movement greater than half range'.)

Gait. The patient's ambulation status was rated as: non-ambulatory or wheelchair dependent; ambulatory, but requiring supervisory assistance; or independently ambulatory with or without gait aids.

Gross motor performance. In total, 16 features of gross motor performance were evaluated via a six-point scale (Fig. 2.2). The patient's total score was divided by 16 and he or she was then described as belonging to one of six levels. Level one, for instance, consisted of patients who were unable to move without assistance, while 'level two patients' could perform the movements only with a great deal of assistance; the assistance required decreased through

_____
* Measures of the reliability of the assessment are currently under study as are further measures of its validity.

GROSS MOTOR PERFORMANCE

Grading Key:
1. Unable to move
2. Able to move with a great deal of assistance
3. Able to move with light assistance
4. Able to move with supervision
5. Able to move independently
6. Able to move normally

Score A* D**
- Supine – R – prone
- Supine – L – prone
- Prone – R – supine
- Prone – L – supine
- Supine – R – sitting
- Supine – L – sitting
- Supine – 4-point kneel
- Crawling

Score A D
- 4-point kneel – kneel stand
- Kneel walking
- Kneel stand - 1/2 kneel stand (R)
- Kneel stand - 1/2 kneel stand (L)
- Bed to chair
- Chair to bed
- Floor to standing
- Standing to floor

Total
Divided by 16
Score

*A = on admission
**D = on discharge

Fig. 2.2 Evaluation form for gross motor performance (from Physiotherapy Canada 34: 77–84, 1982).

to level six, at which point patients were able to move in a relatively normal manner.

Sensation. Not all patients could be reliably tested for sensory status because of disorders in communication or mentation; in total, 258 patients were evaluated (Fig. 2.3). The format for scoring was similar to that of the gross motor performance assessment. Patients with a score of less than 50% were described as being impaired, while those with 50% or more were specified as being mildly impaired or functionally normal. One hundred and sixteen patients had impaired sensation, while 142 were depicted as 'normal'.

Severity of paralysis. Because the severity of the paralysis, or the presence of hemiplegia versus hemiparesis, had been described as a prognostic indicator affecting many aspects of outcome, it seemed logical that it might also be a prime indicator of physical recovery

GROSS SENSATION

Grading Key:
1. severely impaired or absent
2. moderately impaired
3. slightly impaired
4. normal

UNABLE TO TEST ☐ Probably decreased ☐
Probably intact ☐
Uncertain ☐

or

PROPRIOCEPTION and SUPERFICIAL SENSATION

	Position score A* D**		Touch A D	Pain A D
Shoulder	☐☐	Upper arm	☐☐	☐☐
Elbow	☐☐	Forearm	☐☐	☐☐
Pronation/Supination	☐☐	Fingers	☐☐	☐☐
Wrist	☐☐	Thigh	☐☐	☐☐
Fingers	☐☐	Foreleg	☐☐	☐☐
Hip	☐☐	Foot	☐☐	☐☐
Knee	☐☐			
Ankle	☐☐			
			Total	☐☐
			Divided by 20	
			Score	☐☐

*A = on admission
**D = on discharge

Fig. 2.3 Evaluation form for gross sensation (from Physiotherapy Canada 34: 77–84, 1982).

potential. Patients therefore were described as being (a) hemiplegic, that is, possessing no voluntary movement of the arm or leg without facilitation (stages of motor recovery 1 and 2); (b) hemiparetic, that is, having voluntary, but not normal, movement of the affected arm or leg (stages 3 to 5); or (c) normal, that is having movement of the arm and leg with normal timing and coordination (stage 6). One hundred and forty two patients were found to be hemiplegic, 170 hemiparetic and 23 normal.

Shoulder pain. Of 110 patients assessed for shoulder pain at the time of admission, 22 had no complaints while 32 complained of mild and 56 moderate to severe pain.

Mean and standard deviation scores at time of admission and discharge for those characteristics for which such measures are appropriate are summarized in Table 2.1.

Data analysis

Chi square analysis. To describe the magnitude of recovery and to determine the value of the prognostic indicators (components one and two of the study), the data from the 223 patients were subjected to analysis although the data on the perceptual and sensory status of patients were incomplete. In addition, certain other patients were excluded from some of the analysis: patients with bilateral involvement, for instance, were excluded from an analysis of the effect of side of involvement (right versus left), and patients already at the top of the scale (that is, those who could show no further improvement) were excluded when the amount of improvement was the dependent variable.

Measures of physical status, that is, the stage of motor recovery of the arm and leg, the gait level and the gross motor performance, were analyzed to provide a profile of the magnitude of recovery during the rehabilitation period. Following this analysis, the six patient characteristics (sensation, perception, severity of hemiplegia, age, time post-stroke, and the side of hemiplegia) were considered for their value as prognostic indicators.

Table 2.1 Patient characteristics at the time of admission and discharge.

Variable	Admission Score (mean ± SD)	Discharge score (mean ± AD)	No. of patients
Age	63 ± 12	—*	335
Aphasia	75.5 ± 32	—	334
Perception	69.5 ± 26	73.0 ± 19	276
Sensation	2.58 ± 1.15	2.82 ± 1.11	258
Mental status	3.15 ± 0.85	—	111
ADL	20.52 ± 7.99	23.84 ± 4.77	112
Locomotion	1.45 ± 1.20	2.64 ± 1.25	112
Bladder	3.13 ± 0.99	—	112
Stage of arm	2.72 ± 1.67	3.14 ± 1.71	332
Stage of leg	3.21 ± 1.62	3.79 ± 1.59	333
Gross motor	3.13 ± 1.39	4.0 ± 1.49	333
Postural control	4.44 ± 0.86	4.89 ± 32.38	111
Gait	1.60 ± 1.04	2.31 ± 1.03	335
Gait aids	—*	2.52 ± 1.60	50
Speed	—	19.69 ± 12.1	50
Shoulder pain	1.27 ± .81	1.30 ± .79	107

* information not included in analyses.

To determine whether a systematic relationship existed between each measure of physical status and each possible predictive variable, a simple chi-square (x^2) analysis (a comparison of the cell frequencies between each pair of variables) was performed.

Regression analysis. To identify the predictive value of the various patient characteristics (component three of the study), the data from the 335 patients were analyzed. This was done in order to determine the relationship between the 14 dependent or outcome variables of sensori-motor performance and the set of 23 independent or criterion variables. The type of multivariate analysis used in this component of the study, was multiple regression. 'This is a general statistical technique through which one can analyze relationships between a dependent or criterion variable and a set of independent or predictor variables' (Kim & Kohout, 1975, p 321).

The dependent or criterion variables were outcomes that followed stroke rehabilitation, while the independent or predictor variables were patient characteristics present at the time of admission for rehabilitation. The data were analyzed using SPSS multiple regression with forward (stepwise) inclusion. Numerical values were assigned to all characteristics. A set of dummy variables was 'created' for all variables for which the level of measurement was nominal. Characteristics for which dummy variables were 'created' included gender, side of hemiplegia, handedness, artery involved and discharge disposition. For all other variables it was assumed that the level of measurement was ordinal, interval or ratio. The values assigned to variables considered in the regression equations are listed in Table 2.2.

Prospective study. The purpose of the prospective study was to test the accuracy (predictive validity) of the equations developed. Seven of the 11 equations generated from the regression analysis were placed on the clinical assessment form in November, 1982. The seven equations included stage of recovery of the arm, leg and postural control; gross motor performance; sensation; gait and number of gait aids. Results comparing predicted outcomes with actual outcomes (the actual outcomes were based on discharge scores) were available for analysis from a population of 20 patients. A chi square analysis with measures of diagonal agreement, chance agreement and agreement beyond chance (i.e., Cohen's Kappa) comparing predicted and actual outcomes of these 20 patients was performed.

Variable	Value	Variable	Value
Age	Years	ADL (Schoening, 1968; SKI, 1978)	0 = severe 28 = normal
Sex*	0 = male 1 = female	Locomotion and bladder (Schoening, 1968; SKI, 1978)	0 = severe 4 = normal
Side of hemiplegia*	0 = right 1 = left 2 = bilateral	Arm, leg, gross motor and postural control	1 = severe 6 = normal
Handedness*	0 = right 1 = left	Length of stay, weeks from onset to admission	Weeks
Aphasia (Porch, 1972)**, perception (OSOT, undated)	1 = severe 100 = normal	Gait	1 = wheelchair 2 = supervised 3 = normal
Sensation	1 = absent 2 = severely impaired 3 = mildly impaired 4 = normal	Gait aids	1 = quad cane and brace 2 = cane and brace 3 = quad cane 4 = cane 5 = none
Mental status (Pfeiffer, 1975)	1 = severe 4 = normal	Speed of walk	Meters per minute
Family	1 = none 2 = non supportive 3 = supportive	Shoulder pain	0 = moderate to severe 1 = mild 3 = none
Artery*	1 = middle cerebral 2 = other	Discharge disposition*	0 = home 1 = institution
Complications	No. of major complications		
CTT scan	1 = haemorrhage 2 = infarction 3 = normal		

* indicates nominal data for which dummy tables were generated   **assessment reference

Results

Magnitude of recovery

All aspects of the physical status of the patients (the stages of recovery of the arm and leg, the gait level and the level of gross performance) improved significantly during the patients' stay in the rehabilitation centre (Fig. 2.4).

Few patients regained arm function, however. At the time of admission, 24 patients had coordinated arm movements (stage 6) and 20 had individual joint movements but were still classed as clumsy (stage 5), for a total of 44 patients or 20% of the study's population. By the time of discharge, these numbers had changed to 31 in stage 6 and 25 in stage 5, for a total of 56 patients or 25%. Nevertheless, only 5% of the population had gained sufficient motor recovery during the rehabilitative stay to perform individual joint movements of the involved arm—a prerequisite of function.

In comparison to the 5% who regained arm function, 22% benefited from an improved voluntary movement of the leg sufficient for ambulation (that is, they moved from stages 1 and 2 to stages 3 to 6).

The greatest gains were seen in the gait status. At the time of admission, 53 patients were already ambulatory (24%); at discharge 110 walked independently while 46 walked with supervision—a total of 156 patients or 70%. These changes resulted in 46% of the total population of the study's patients reambulating during rehabilitation.

At the time of admission, 42 patients (19%) were independent in gross motor performance, that is, they obtained a mean score of five or six in activities such as rolling, sitting, knee standing and transferring to and from the floor. By the time of discharge, this noumber had expanded to 95 patients or a change of 24%

These four measures of change in the physical status of patients along with information on prognostic indicators can serve as general indicators of what might be expected at the end of a rehabilitation period.

Prognostic indicators

Of the six characteristics investigated (sensation, perception, severity of hemiplegia, age, length of time from onset of stroke to admission to the rehabilitation centre, and the side of hemiplegia), only the side of hemiplegia failed to relate significantly to outcome. The specific relationships between outcome and patient characteristics are as follows.

Reambulation. The characteristic that showed the closest relationship to a patient's potential for reambulation was found to be the length of time post-stroke prior to admittance. Patients admitted to the rehabilitation centre more than 12 weeks after the onset of their stroke were significantly less likely to walk again than were their counterparts admitted earlier (Table 2.3). Other factors adversely affecting the potential for reambulation were hemiplegia (Table 2.4), involved perception (Tables 2.5), advanced age (Table 2.6) and loss of sensation (Table 2.7).

Improved gross motor performance. The potential for improving gross motor performance, like that of ambulation, was significantly reduced in patients more than 12 weeks post-stroke (Table 2.3). Advanced age (Table 2.6) and a complete hemiplegia (Table 2.4) also correlated with less improvement in gross motor performance.

Improved stage of motor recovery. Fewer factors affected the recovery potential of the leg. Again, time post-stroke showed the highest predictive value (Table 2.3), and only advanced age added to the picture by adversely affecting outcome (Table 2.6). None of the variables investigated affected outcome of the arm. It should be noted, however, that 19 patients with normal sensation were admitted with a stage 6 arm while only one patient with involved sensation had such a high level of motor function. This information suggests that patients with normal sensation recover motor control of the arm earlier than those with involved sensation (Table 2.7).

The finding that the side of hemiplegia did not relate significantly to outcome suggests that the left-sided individual with hemiplegia can be expected to perform about as well as the individual with a right hemiplegia (Table 2.8). This information, along with the findings documented in Table 2.5, suggest that it is the presence or absence of a perceptual deficit rather than the side of the hemiplegia *per se* that affects recovery.

Taken by themselves, measures of the magnitude of recovery and a description of the relationship between the prognostic indicators and the sensori-motor recovery can serve only as general indicators of what might be expected at the end of a rehabilitation period. To make a more precise prediction of expected changes in sensori-motor recovery, the more complex and subtle interactions of the several factors simultaneously must also be considered.

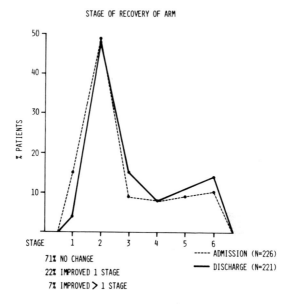

STAGE OF RECOVERY OF ARM

71% NO CHANGE
22% IMPROVED 1 STAGE
7% IMPROVED > 1 STAGE

---- ADMISSION (N=226)
—— DISCHARGE (N=221)

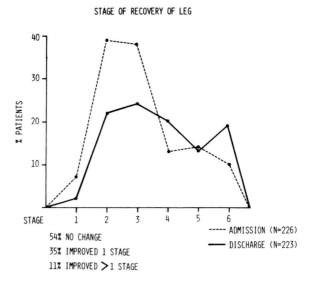

STAGE OF RECOVERY OF LEG

54% NO CHANGE
35% IMPROVED 1 STAGE
11% IMPROVED > 1 STAGE

---- ADMISSION (N=226)
—— DISCHARGE (N=223)

Fig. 2.4 Status of the arm, leg, gait and gross motor performance of 223 stroke patients at the time of admission to and discharge from treatment in a rehabilitation centre. The broken line indicates the status at the of admission; the solid line at the time of discharge. The stages refer to the Brunnstrom stages of recovery; the levels of gait refer to wheelchair dependent (W/C), supervised gait

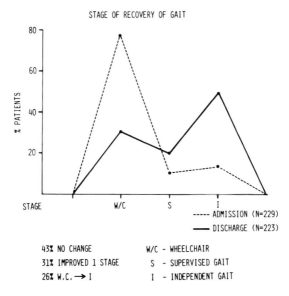

STAGE OF RECOVERY OF GAIT

43% NO CHANGE	W/C - WHEELCHAIR
31% IMPROVED 1 STAGE	S - SUPERVISED GAIT
26% W.C. → I	I - INDEPENDENT GAIT

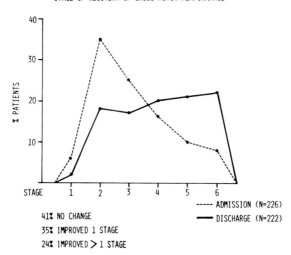

STAGE OF RECOVERY OF GROSS MOTOR PERFORMANCE

41% NO CHANGE
35% IMPROVED 1 STAGE
24% IMPROVED > 1 STAGE

(S) and independent gait (I); and the levels of gross motor performance correspond to the range from total dependence (1) to normal coordinated movement (6). Significant recovery occurred during rehabilitation in all parameters: arm $x^2 = 17.06$, $p = 0.004$; leg $x^2 = 28.83$, $p < 0.0001$; gait $x^2 = 98.88$, $p < 0.0001$; gross motor performance $x^2 = 38.64$, $p < 0.0001$ (from Physiotherapy Canada 34: 77–84, 1982).

Table 2.3 Comparison of the amount of recovery in the arm, leg, gait and gross motor performance of stroke patients up to and after 12 weeks (N = 223)

	Cases < 12 weeks	Cases > 12 weeks
Gait		
no improvement	38 (16)*	30 (13)
1 level of improvement	56	12
2 or more levels of improvement	50	8
	$x^2 = 18.66$	$p < 0.0001$
Gross motor performance		
no improvement	43 (15)	30 (4)
1 level of improvement	56	21
2 or more levels of improvement	46	8
	$x^2 = 10.59$	$p = 0.005$
Leg		
no improvement	58 (17)	39 (5)
1 stage of improvement	60	18
2 or more stages of improvement	25	1
	$x^2 = 15.29$	$p = 0.0005$
Arm		
no improvement	89 (18)	44 (5)
1 stage of improvement	36	12
2 or more stages of improvement	17	2
	$x^2 = 4.60$	$p = 0.100$

* The figures in parentheses represent the number of patients excluded from the calculations because they had no deficit in that particular feature at the time of admission (from Physiotherapy Canada 34: 77–84, 1982).

Table 2.4 Comparison of the amount of recovery in the arm, leg, gait and gross motor performance of stroke patients with hemiplegia and hemiparesis (N = 208)

	Cases with hemiplegia	Cases with hemiparesis
Gait		
no improvement	47 (1)*	22 (17)
1 level of improvement	23	42
2 or more levels of improvement	26	30
	$x^2 = 14.88$	$p = 0.0006$
Gross motor performance		
no improvement	40 (0)	32 (10)
1 level of improvement	26	47
2 or more levels of improvement	31	22
	$x^2 = 8.38$	$p = 0.015$
Leg		
no improvement	45 (0)	54 (7)
1 stage of improvement	35	43
2 or more stages of improvement	17	7
	$x^2 = 5.57$	$p = 0.062$
Arm		
no improvement	69 (0)	67 (8)
1 stage of improvement	23	25
2 or more stages of improvement	5	11
	$x^2 = 2.19$	$p = 0.335$

* The figures in parentheses represent the number of patients excluded from the calculations because they had no deficit in that particular feature at the time of admission (from Physiotherapy Canada 34: 77–84, 1982).

Table 2.5 Comparison of the amount of recovery in the arm, leg, gait and gross motor performance of stroke patients with and without perceptual involvement (N = 166)

	Cases with: perceptual involvement	normal perception
Gait		
no improvement	39 (5)★	13 (14)
1 level of improvement	29	17
2 or more levels of improvement	21	28
	$x^2 = 11.09$	$p = 0.004$
Gross motor performance		
no improvement	31 (4)	22 (12)
1 level of improvement	40	20
2 or more levels of improvement	19	18
	$x^2 = 2.32$	$p = 0.314$
Leg		
no improvement	46 (5)	27 (11)
1 stage of improvement	35	24
2 or more stages of improvement	8	10
	$x^2 = 2.06$	$p = 0.356$
Arm		
no improvement	62 (4)	36 (12)
1 stage of improvement	17	17
2 or more stages of improvement	10	7
	$x^2 = 1.97$	$p = 0.373$

★ The figures in parentheses represent the number of patients excluded from the calculations because they had no deficit in that particular feature at the time of admission (from Physiotherapy Canada 34: 77–84, 1982)

Table 2.6 Comparison of the amount of recovery in the arm, leg, gait and gross motor performance between stroke patients older than 55 years and those 55 years of age and younger (N = 223)

	Cases ⩽ 55 years	Cases > 55 years
Gait		
no improvement	10 (10)★	58 (19)
1 level of improvement	19	49
2 or more levels of improvement	23	35
	$x^2 = 10.00$	$p = 0.007$
Gross motor performance		
no improvement	13 (6)	60 (3)
1 level of improvement	20	57
2 or more levels of improvement	23	31
	$x^2 = 9.71$	$p = 0.008$
Leg		
no improvement	20 (4)	77 (18)
1 stage of improvement	27	51
2 or more stages of improvement	11	15
	$x^2 = 6.76$	$p = 0.034$
Arm		
no improvement	35 (6)	98 (17)
1 stage of improvement	14	34
2 or more stages of improvement	7	12
	$x^2 = 0.96$	$p = 0.620$

★ The figures in parentheses represent the number of patients excluded from the calculations because they had no deficit in that particular feature at the time of admission. (from Physiotherapy Canada, 34: 77–84, 1982)

Table 2.7 Comparison of the amount of recovery in the arm, leg, gait and gross motor performance of stroke patients with and without sensory involvement (N = 174)

	Cases with sensory involvement	Cases with normal sensation
Gait		
no improvement	31 (2)★	15 (21)
1 level of improvement	21	32
2 or more levels of improvement	25	27
	$x^2 = 7.87$	$p = 0.020$
Gross motor performance		
no improvement	27 (1)	26 (16)
1 level of improvement	29	33
2 or more levels of improvement	22	20
	$x^2 = 0.37$	$p = 0.833$
Leg		
no improvement	34 (1)	36 (17)
1 stage of improvement	35	30
2 or more stages of improvement	9	12
	$x^2 = 0.87$	$p = 0.647$
Arm		
no improvement	57 (1)	43 (19)
1 stage of improvement	14	23
2 or more stages of improvement	7	10
	$x^2 = 4.65$	$p = 0.098$

★ The figures in parentheses represent the number of patients excluded from the calculations because they had no deficit in that particular feature at the time of admission (from Physiotherapy Canada 34: 77–84, 1982)

Table 2.8 Comparison of the amount of recovery in the arm, leg, gait and gross motor performance of stroke patients with right-sided and left-sided hemiplegia (N = 215)

	Cases with right-sided hemiplegia	Cases with left-sided hemiplegia
Gait		
no imporvement	39 (15)★	47 (12)
1 level of improvement	35	41
2 or more levels of improvement	8	18
	$x^2 = 2.03$	$p = 0.362$
Gross motor performance		
no improvement	28 (10)	41 (6)
1 level of improvement	34	42
2 or more levels of improvement	25	29
	$x^2 = 0.45$	$p = 0.797$
Leg		
no improvement	43 (11)	51 (8)
1 level of improvement	35	41
2 or more stages of improvement	8	18
	$x^2 = 2.09$	$p = 0.351$
Arm		
no improvement	51 (14)	77 (6)
1 stage of improvement	26	22
2 or more stages of improvement	6	13
	$x^2 = 3.97$	$p = 0.137$

★ The figures in parentheses represent the number of patients excluded from the calculations because they had no deficit in that particular feature at the time of admission (from Physiotherapy Canada 34: 77–84, 1982)

Predictions

The criterion for deciding that an equation would be clinically useful for predicting the level of sensori-motor recovery following rehabilitation was arbitrarily established, that is, the predictive variables in the equations had to explain at least 50% of the variance in outcome. This can be evaluated by examining the square of the multiple correlation (i.e., R^2). For purpose of comprehension, the multiple correlation (i.e., R) can be interpreted in the same way as is a simple correlation (i.e., r), where a correlation coefficient provides an easy means for comparing the strength of the relationship between two pairs of variables with zero indicating no relationship and $+1.0$ or -1.0 indicating a perfect linear relationship.

In all, 11 of the 14 equations generated through regression analysis were found to be clinically useful. This included equations for predicting the outcome of ADL, stage of the arm, stage of the leg, postural control, gross motor performance, sensation, perception, gait, number of gait aids, gait speed and shoulder pain (Table 2.9).

Only three of the equations failed to be clinically useful, that is, less than 50% of the outcome variance for discharge disposition, length of stay and locomotion on the Kenny scale could be

Table 2.9   Clinically useful predictive equations ($R^2 > 0.50$)

Predicted discharge status $\pm$ standard error

ADL $\pm$ 3.23 = 12.57 + 2.58 B* + 0.87 GM + 1.07 H (R^2 = 0.55, N = 112)
Arm $\pm$ 0.76 = 0.41 + 0.86 A + 0.27 L − 0.01 W (R^2 = 0.81, N = 332)
Leg $\pm$ 0.77 = 1.50 + 0.86 L − 0.01 W − 0.01 Ag (R^2 = 0.77, N = 332)
Postural control $\pm$ 0.60 = 1.04 + 0.86 PC (R^2 = 0.73, N = 110)
Gross motor $\pm$ 0.93 = 2.65 + 0.68 GM − 0.02 Ag + 0.13 L − 0.01 W (R^2 = 0.61, N = 332)
Sensation $\pm$ 0.39 = 0.05 + 0.89 S + 0.14 MS (R^2 = 0.87, N = 88)
Perception $\pm$ 10.25 = 0.64 + 0.03 P + 0.53 L (R^2 = 0.73, N = 109)
Gait $\pm$ 0.67 = 1.77 + 0.66 G + 0.12 GM − 0.01 Ag − 0.01 W (R^2 = 0.59, N = 332)
Gait aids $\pm$ 1.13 = 0.78 + 0.92 L − 0.13 LS − 0.36 C (R^2 = 0.53, N = 50)
Gait speed × 60 $\pm$ 0.13 = 0.13 L − 1.6 Sx − 0.12 (R^2 0.59, N = 50)
Shoulder pain $\pm$ 0.53 − 0.63 SP + 0.01 PC + 0.01 P − 0.42 (R^2 = 0.56, N = 107)

---

* Letters in equations refer to status on admission.

A = stage of arm	LS = length of stay
Ag = age	MS = mental status
B = bladder and bowel	P = perception
C = number of major complications	PC = postural control
G = gait	S = sensation
GM = gross motor performance	SP = shoulder pain
H = side of hemiplegia	Sx = gender
L = stage of leg	W = weeks from onset to admission

predicted (Table 2.10). However, in all three cases patient characteristics that made a statistically significant contribution to predicting these outcomes were identified (Table 2.10).

In order to ascertain the relative predictive value of each of the 23 patient characteristics, the number of equations in which each appeared was counted. Stage of recovery of the leg was found to be the most important predictive variable as it appeared in seven of 14 equations. It was followed in importance by weeks post stroke, which appeared in six equations, and gross motor performance, which appeared in four. Five variables, that is, ADL, aphasia, artery involved, CTT scan and handedness were not included in any of the predictive equations (Table 2.11).

Prospective study

Table 2.12 shows the results of the chi square analysis, comparing the seven predicted outcomes with the actual outcomes. In all cases, outcomes had been predicted at a statistically significant level (i.e., $p < 0.05$).

In addition, the agreement beyond chance (Cohen's Kappa) was acceptably high ($K \geqslant 0.70$) except for the prediction of postural control and gait status. However, if the score predicting gait status was combined with that for predicting the number of gait aids, a high value for agreement beyond chance also was available for predicting gait.

Discussion

This study, along with the work of other authors, suggests that many aspects of post-stroke, sensori-motor recovery can be reliably

Table 2.10 Outcomes for which significant* predictive variables were identified but equations failed to be of clinical use ($R^2 < 0.50$) (From Physiotherapy Canada 36: 313–320, 1984)

Outcome	Predictive variables	
Discharge disposition	urinary continence, family support	($R^2 = 0.07$, N = 107)
Length of stay	stage of arm, stage of leg, gross motor performance and weeks post stroke	($R^2 = 0.19$, N = 332)
Kenny locomotion	locomotion and weeks post stroke	($R^2 = 0.48$, N = 112)

    * $p < 0.05$ two tailed

Table 2.11 Rank order of the 23 patient characteristics as predictors of outcome

No. of outcomes each characteristic played a significant role in predicting	Characteristic
7	stage of leg
6	weeks post stroke
4	gross motor performance
3	age
2	perception
	postural control
	stage of arm
	urinary continence
1	complications
	family
	gait
	length of stay
	locomotion
	mental status
	sensation
	sex
	shoulder pain
	side of hemiplegia
0	ADL
	aphasia
	artery
	CTT scan*
	handedness

* CTT scans were available on a small number of patients (N = 25)

predicted at the outset of an active rehabilitation program. These aspects include such features as discharge disposition, length of stay, general rehabilitation and ADL potential, as well as the recovery of the arm, leg, postural control, gross motor perform-ance, sensation and gait. It would appear that therapists are justi-fied in collecting information on a large number of patient characteristics at the time of admission as many of these need to be considered in predicting the outcome of these various aspects of recovery.

Not all studies agree on the specific patient characteristics that offer the best predictive value. This could be explained by differ-ences in the list of characteristics investigated, the way in which the characteristics were measured and whether regression analysis had been used. It is important to note that regression analysis controls for confounding factors while evaluating the contribution of a specific variable. As well, it allows for the deletion of independent variables that do not add substantially to prediction accuracy (Kim & Kohout, 1975, p. 321).

Table 2.12 Predictive validity of equations in determining outcomes: a prospective analysis (N = 20) (From Physiotherapy Canada 36: 313–320, 1984)

Outcome	χ^2 Value (df)	Significance level	Diagonal agreement	Chance agreement	Cohen's kappa
Arm	65.7 (25)	$p < 0.001$	0.95	0.62	0.87
Leg	32.2 (16)	$p < 0.01$	0.86	0.55	0.70
Postural control	16.0 (9)	$p = 0.001$	0.85	0.59	0.64
Gross motor	40.3 (16)	$p < 0.001$	0.89	0.60	0.72
Sensation	17.7 (1)	$p = .001$	0.92	0.70	0.72
Gait	12.2 (4)	$p < 0.05$	0.75	0.57	0.42
Gait plus aids*	18.3 (4)	$p = 0.001$	0.88	0.53	0.73
Gait aids	44.6 (16)	$p = .001$	0.94	0.59	0.85

* If gait aids score was combined with gait score in predicting ambulation status.

Recovery magnitude

There is general agreement that approximately 4 to 5% of the population will regain the functional use of the upper extremity with approximately 40 to 60% regaining voluntary motion. Similarly, there is general agreement about the number of patients who will reambulate. The finding that 70% of patients included in this study walked at the time of discharge is consistent with the findings of others who reported that 61 to 85% of surviving stroke patients could be expected to walk again.

Discharge disposition

The list of patient characteristics found to correlate with discharge disposition includes urinary incontinence, family support, severity of the weakness, time from onset, gait status and family income. Family income had not been included in the list of independent variables used in regression analysis. From the above list only urinary incontinence and family support appeared in the regression equation.

Length of stay

Patient characteristics found to correlate with length of stay include some measure of the severity of the motor involvement* (e.g. stage of recovery of the arm and leg), gait, status, gross motor performance and weeks post onset, as well as those independent variables identified by Ben-Yishay et al (1970), consisting of a clinical demographic set of six variables, a sensory motor set of three variables, the WAIS and the Bender-Gestalt. From this list of variables only gait status failed to appear in a regression equation.

Functional status

Self-care. Two variables emerged as highly significant in the prediction of ADL status. These were urinary incontinence and some measure of the severity of the weakness (strength of hip extensors, sitting or standing balance, motor deficit in the arm or gross motor performance). Four additional variables were identified by more than one study as important; these included time since

---

* Feigenson et al (1977) included hemiparesis in the presence of severe organic mental syndrome, severe perceptual dysfunction or poor motivation.

onset, previous CVA, WAIS and age. Twenty variables were found to have predictive value in one of the studies. These were gender, side of hemiplegia, hemianopsia, sensation, socioeconomic factors (educational level, marital status, occupational rating or source of income), ADL score on admission, part B of the trail making test, Bender-Gestalt, elevated systolic blood pressure, decubitus ulcers and tongue protrusion.

Ambulation. The demographic and psychometric measures identified by Ben-Yishay et al (1970), as well as ambulation status on admission, gross motor performance, age, time since onset and severity of the motor involvement, were all found to aid in predicting the quality of ambulation. All of these variables were included in a regression equation.

Other sensori-motor outcomes. Equations for predicting recovery in the hemiplegic arm and leg, postural control, gross motor performance, sensation, perception, gait aids, gait speed and shoulder pain have been identified. The independent variables that aided significantly in predicting these items are listed in Table 2.9.

Although sensori-motor outcomes can be predicted to a large extent with the equations identified to date, part of the variance in outcomes still cannot be explained. Both improved measurement of patient characteristics and inclusion of additional characteristics such as motivation, could help in this regard.

For some of the variables analyzed by this study a more complete set of data is required. For example, CTT scan results from a larger population may have shown that this measure of neurological involvement explains a significant amount of variance in outcome as is suggested by the work of others (Lundgren et al, 1982; Soderstron et al, 1981).

Regression analysis is not ideally suited for the analysis of ordinal data. This may account for unexplained variance. It has been observed that patients with initial assessment scores that are very low, generally do more poorly than predicted, while those with high scores at the time of initial assessment do better. This supports the notion that the method of quantifying the patient characteristics needs refinement (Michaels, 1983).

To date, the equations available cannot be generalized to predict outcomes for the stroke population at large as they came from a population of patients requiring intensive inpatient rehabilitation. It would be valuable to develop equations from a population of stroke patients with acute involvement.

The results of this study provide further evidence (Fugl-Meyer et al, 1975; Clarke et al, 1983) of the validity of the Brunnstrom method of staging the recovery of the arm and leg. It should be noted that stage of recovery of the leg plays a part in predicting more aspects of of recovery than does any other single characteristic investigated in this study, ranking ahead of such important variables as weeks post stroke and age, while the stage of recovery of the arm ranks ahead of such commonly noted features as side of hemiplegia, mental status and sensation. Wade et al (1983) also found that a motor deficit in the arm was second only to urinary incontinence in predicting functional outcome.

Conclusions

This study provides physical therapists with equations found to be clinically useful for predicting the level of sensori-motor recovery that can be expected following stroke rehabilitation. Outcomes that can be predicted include ADL, stage of the arm, stage of the leg, postural control, gross motor performance, sensation, perception, gait, gait aids, gait speed and shoulder pain.

From the list of patient characteristics commonly assessed at time of admission to rehabilitation, those which play a significant role in predicting outcomes are identified. Ranking these from most to least important they include stage of leg, weeks post stroke, gross motor performance, age, perception, postural control, stage of the arm, urinary continency, major medical complications, family support, gait, length of stay, locomotion, mental status, sensation, gender, shoulder pain and side of hemiplegia. Five characteristics commonly assessed play no role in predicting the outcomes investigated. These are ADL, aphasia, artery involved, CTT scan and handedness. This finding relative to the CTT scan should be interpreted guardedly.

Characteristics that had not been evaluated for their prognostic significance by this study but warrant consideration in future work fall into four categories: pathologic signs and symptoms, pertinent history, socioeconomic and psychometric measures. Included in the list of patholic signs and symptoms are hemianopsia, elevated systolic blood pressure, decubitus ulcers and tongue protrusion. The important prognostic feature of the medical history appears to be a previous CVA. Included in the list of socioeconomic measures is the amount and source of family income, educational level, marital status, motivation and occupational rating. The psychometric measures identified include the WAIS, the Bender-Gestalt, part B of the trail making test, the Purdue and two point discrimination.

The knowledge gained from studies such as these can be applied to design more effective and efficient treatment programmes and thus can be beneficial in evaluating quality of care and programme effectiveness. The ability to judge which stroke survivors might be expected to regain functional recovery of, for example, the hemiplegic arm would determine the choice of physiotherapy programme appropriate to the expected outcome. Intensive rehabilitation programmes should be based on the prospect of individual patients benefiting from them. Costly programmes with little or no rehabilitative effect are recognized as poor rehabilitative practice.

ACKNOWLEDGEMENT

Some of the material in this chapter was previously published in two articles in *Physiotherapy Canada*. The first article is entitled *Recovery of motor function following stroke: profile and predictors*, Vol. 34, no. 2, pages 77–84, 1982. The second article is entitled *Predicting sensorimotor recovery following stroke rehabilitation*, Vol. 36, no. 6, pages 313–320, 1984. This material is reprinted with permission of the editor of *Physiotherapy Canada*.

REFERENCES

Adams G F, McComb S G 1953 Assessment and prognosis in hemiplegia. Lancet ii: 266–269

Anderson E K 1967 The significance of parietal lobes in hemiplegia. Hawaii Medical Journal 27: 141–145

Anderson T P, Bourestom N, Greenberg F R, Hildyard V G 1974 Predictive factors in stroke rehabilitation. Archives of Physical Medicine and Rehabilitation 55: 545–553

Bard G, Hirschberg G G 1965 Recovery of voluntary motion in upper extremity following hemiplegia. Archives of Physical Medical and Rehabilitation 46: 567–572

Ben-Yishay Y, Gertsman L, Diller L, Haas A 1970 Prediction of rehabilitation outcomes from psychometric parameters in left hemiplegics. Journal of Consulting and Clinical Psychology 34: 436–441

Bourestom N C, Howard M T 1968 Behavioral correlates of recovery in self-care in hemiplegic patients. Archives of Physical Medical and Rehabilitation 49: 449–454

Brunnstrom S 1970 Movement therapy in hemiplegia. Harper and Row, New York

Clarke B, Gowland C, Brandstater M, De Bruin H 1983 A re-evaluation of the Brunnstrom assessment of motor recovery of the lower limb. Physiotherapy Canada 35: 207–211

Elinson J 1974 Methods of health care evaluation. In: Sackett D L, Baskin M S (eds) Oral presentation, 3rd edn. McMaster University, Hamilton

Feigenson J S, McDowell F H, Meese P, McCarthy M L, Greenburg S D 1977 Factors influencing outcome and length of stay in a stroke rehabilitation unit. Stroke 8: 651–662

Fugl-Meyer A R, Jaasko L, Layman I, Olsson S, Steglind S 1975 The post-stroke hemiplegic patient: a method of evaluation of physical performance. Scandinavian Journal of Rehabilitation Medicine 7: 13–31

Gersten J W 1975 Rehabilitation potential. In: Licht S (ed) Stroke and its rehabilitation. Licht, New Haven, CT, pp 435–471

Joshi J, Singh N, Varma S K 1974 Residual motor deficits in adult hemiplegic patients. Proceedings: World Conference for Physical Therapy, Seventh International Congress, Montreal, Quebec

Kim J O, Kohout F J 1975 Multiple regressional analysis; subprogram regression. In: Nie N H, Hull C H, Jenkins J G, Steinbrenner K, Bent D (eds) Statistical package for the social sciences, 2nd edn. McGraw-Hill, New York

Lehmann J F, DeLateur B J, Fowler R S, Warren C G, Arnhold R, Schertzer G et al 1975 Stroke rehabilitation: outcome and prediction. Archives of Physical Medicine and Rehabilitation 56: 383–389

Lorenze E J, Cancro R 1962 Dysfunction in visual perception with hemiplegia: its relation to activities of daily living. Archives of Physical Medicine and Rehabilitation 43: 524–517

Lundgren J, Flodstrom K, Sjogren K, Liljequist B, Fugl-Meyer A R 1982 Sight of brain lesion and functional capacity in rehabilitated hemiplegics. Scandinavian Journal of Rehabilitation Medicine 14: 141–143

MacLeod R D M, Williamson J 1972 Problems of stroke assessment and rehabilitation. Scottish Medical Journal 12: 384–389

Michaels E 1983 Measurement in physical therapy: on the rules of assigning numerals to observations. Physical Therapy 63: 209–215

Mills V M, DiGenio M 1983 Functional differences in patients with left or right cerebrovascular accidents. Physical Therapy 63: 481–488

Moskowitz E, Lightbody F E M, Freitag N 1972 Long-term follow up of the post-stroke patient. Archives of Physical Medicine and Rehabilitation 53: 167–172

OSOT Study Group on the Brain Damaged Adult undated Manual on perceptual evaluation. Ontario Society of Occupational Therapy, Toranto

Peszczyniski M 1964 Rehabilitation of adult hemiplegic locomotor system. In: Fourth Annual Volume of Physiologic and Experimental Medical Sciences, Calcutta, India

Pfeiffer E 1975 A short portable mental status questionnaire for the assessment of organic brain deficit in elderly patients. Journal of the American Geriatrics Society 23: 434–441

Porch B E 1972 Porch Index of Communicative Ability (PICA): theory, development, administration, scoring, interpretation (2 vols.). Consulting Psychologist Press Inc., California

Schoening H A, Iverson J A 1968 Numerical scoring of self care status; a study of the Kenny self care evaluation. Archives of Physical Medicine and Rehabilitation 49: 221–229

Sister Kenny Institute 1978 Revised Kenny self help evaluation. Sister Kenny Institute, Minneapolis, Minnesota

Soderstrom C E, Ericson K, Mattinger K L, Olivecrona H 1981 Computed tomography and CSF spectrophotometry: diagnosis and prognosis in 300 patients with cerebralvascular disease. Scandinavian Journal of Rehabilitation Medicine 13: 65–71

Steinberg F V 1973 The stroke registry: a prospective method of studying Archives of Physical Medicine and Rehabilitation 54: 31–35

Stern P H, McDowell F, Miller J M, Robinson M 1971 Factors influencing stroke rehabilitation. Stroke 2: 213–218

Torresin W, Gowland C, Hall A 1982 Treatment guidelines for motor recovery in hemiplegic patients: postural control, upper extremities, lower extremities and gait. An internal report, Chedoke Rehabilitation Centre

Wade D T, Skilbeck C E, Langton Hewer R 1983 Predicting Barthel ADL score at six months after an acute stroke. Archives of Physical Medicine and Rehabilitation 64: 24–28

Waylonis G W, Keith M W, Aseff J N 1973 Stroke rehabilitation in a midwestern county. Archives of Physical Medicine and Rehabilitation 54: 151–155

Motor training following stroke

INTRODUCTION

Although stroke rehabilitation has to some extent progressed over the years, the results presented in the literature of what is frequently a lengthy rehabilitation process are generally poor. Walking deficits which require an aid, a relatively unfunctional upper extremity and a general malaise are three common sequelae and appear to be the expected disabilities.

These disabilities may not, however, be necessary. Rather than reflecting solely the effect of brain damage, they may represent an habituation of compensatory movements, a 'learned non-use' (Taub, 1980) of the affected extremities, musculo-skeletal and cardio-pulmonary disuse. These problems may occur through deficiencies in rehabilitation and environmental deprivation.

The fact that the above disabilities are accepted may reflect *negative expectations* about both brain damage and old age. Therapeutic attitudes may have been influenced by negative expectations of the brain's capacity for recovery following a lesion. There is, however, substantial evidence from animal studies (Walsh & Cummins, 1976; Goldberger, 1980; Lynch & Wells, 1980) that the brain is capable of reorganisation and adaptation at the anatomical, biochemical and functional level. Anatomical studies, for example, have shown that nerve cells, dendrites, axons and glia appear to possess considerable capacity for growth in the adult brain (Lynch & Wells, 1980). Experiments with monkeys following cortical ablation procedures, indicate that early mobilisation and functional assistance produce good functional results (Travis & Woolsey, 1952, 1956). Perry (1980) comments that rehabilitation of stroke patients, involving 'early mobilisation and assistance in directing their evolving neuro-control into effective function', results in 'far less devastating (loss of function) than that described by Twitchell and assumed to be inevitable by most clinicians'.

Negative expectations about the capacities of the elderly are also held throughout the health professions. Yet studies (Gibbs, 1960; Dubois, 1975) have shown that elderly non brain-damaged subjects are as capable of learning as younger subjects, although the conditions may have to be different in some respects. Other studies have shown that elderly stroke patients are capable of learning new motor tasks (Halberstam & Zaretsky, 1969). Many of the problems of elderly people are due to disuse but these changes appear to be reversible. Payton (1983) reviews several studies which show that exercise reverses many symptoms of ageing and prevents the effects of disuse.

The environment in which a stroke patient finds himself may provide protection, safety and care, but lack stimulation, challenge and the chance to learn. Animal experiments have shown that both training (Greenough, 1976) and the environment (Walsh & Greenough, 1976; Lynch & Wells, 1980) have an effect upon brain structure. Bennett (1976) found that the cerebral cortex of rats which spent their time in a rich and complex environment was measurably thicker and heavier than other rats. Furthermore, this situation could be reversed if the rats were placed in a relatively impoverished environment. The experimenter suggests that the richer environment provided more opportunity for learning.

It may be that in humans who have had a stroke, an emphasis on motor training in contexts appropriate to everyday life and requiring cognitive effort, in an environment which is conducive to learning, may trigger off in the brain a series of changes which will allow for the re-programming of previously well-learned motor acts. In other words, physiotherapy may provide the framework within which these changes can take place.

For a number of years the authors have been developing a motor training programme which represents a shift away from current physiotherapy models to a motor control-motor learning model. The programme, called 'A Motor Relearning Programme' (MRP) (Carr & Shepherd, 1982), has a theoretical basis in studies of human movement, muscle biology, motor skill learning and motivation, and is also derived from the authors' clinical observation that many stroke patients have the capacity to regain effective motor control if the conditions, that is the training and environmental conditions, are appropriate.

EARLY MOTOR TRAINING

The basis of the motor learning—motor control paradigm is described in The Motor Relearning Programme for Stroke under four headings.

The problem-solving process

This can be divided into five stages: recognition, analysis, decision-making, action-taking and re-evaluation. Accurate analysis of motor function and comparison with the normal is crucial to the motor training process and requires not only an understanding of normal function and good observational ability but also the ability to process this information. The therapist arrives at a solution, having considered the problems in terms of biomechanics, muscle biology and behaviour. There are, for example, many biomechanical studies of walking (Saunders, et al 1953; Winter, 1979; Inman, 1981) which give details of the kinematics and kinetics of walking. *Analysis* of a patient's attempts at walking must take these details into account. The therapist observes the patient walking or attempting to walk and notes the missing or abnormal components in stance and swing phase. This requires not only observation but also a survey of the reasons for particular components being absent or poorly controlled. Acting on this information the therapist *makes a decision* as to which component should be retrained first and how this training could take place (*action-taking*).

> *Example 1. Walking*
> This woman (Fig. 3.1a) is having difficulty controlling her R. knee throughout stance phase. Although her quadriceps is sufficiently controlled in outer and middle range to straighten her knee when she is sitting, sustained activity in the shortened position, sufficient to take her weight and allow the knee to flex a few degrees (a lengthening contraction of the quadriceps) is absent. The therapist, therefore, trains the patient to hold a sustained contraction of the quadriceps in inner range (Fig. 3.1b) and to control the lengthening contraction in a position which enables her to concentrate on this one task (Fig. 3.1c). The patient then stands up and practises stepping forward with the intact L. leg, concentrating on extending the weight-bearing R. hip and controlling the knee (Fig. 3.1d).

This practice of controlling the specific muscle activity then the component as part of the activity itself (walking) gives the patient the opportunity to use her improved motor control to improve her walking ability. Furthermore, she can see the relevance of what she

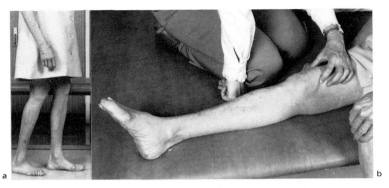

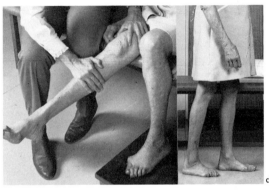

Fig. 3.1 (a) She cannot sustain a quadriceps contraction nor control an eccentric contraction at the appropriate part of stance phase. (b) Training to improve ability to sustain a contraction with the muscle in the shortened position. (c) Training to control an eccentric contraction starting with the muscle in its shortened range. (d) When she steps forward, her performance has improved.

has practised. It also allows the therapist *to re-evaluate* the patient's performance to check on the analysis and the effectiveness of the training.

Contextual significance

It seems probable that, in terms of both motor learning and muscle action, motor training should take place in the functional context in which it is needed (Rasch & Morehouse, 1957; Sale & MacDougall, 1981). Whiting (1980) comments that movement skills will be learned if they are practised 'in the context of the actions they are to subserve'. He also suggests that it is 'not *only* a question of producing co-ordinated movements, but of producing them at will in an *appropriate* context'.

The MRP represents an attempt to train muscle control within specific functional contexts. It is divided into seven sections which together cover a person's everyday motor needs, oro-motor function, upper limb function, standing up and sitting down, balanced sitting and standing, and walking. Each section is divided into four steps. Analysis of function is the *first step*, followed by practice of the missing component *(second step)*, practice of the entire activity *(third step)*, and the *fourth step* includes methods of ensuring that there will be a transference of learning into the patient's daily life.

> *Example 2. Standing up and sitting down*
> Analysis *(Step 1)* of this man's attempts at standing up (Fig. 3.2a) indicates that he has problems with the movement components involved in the activity. For example, he cannot extend his R. hip or knee to gain the normal limb alignment for standing. The therapist explains this to the patient and trains him to activate and sustain a contraction of his gluteus maximus with the muscle at the length which is necessary for standing, in a position in which it is relatively easy for him to practise (Fig. 3.2b). The patient receives verbal feedback from the therapist and manual guidance, so his attempts at muscle control are monitored *(Step 2)*. Practice of this component is followed immediately by practice of standing up again with the performance monitored by the therapist, with emphasis on ensuring that weight is taken through his right leg, and on gaining the necessary limb alignment *(Step 3)*. Figure 3.2c illustrates the improvement in hip alignment and in knee position. Although the quadriceps may not yet be able to contract with sufficient control in its inner range to control a straight knee position for the stance phase of walking, the improved limb alignment allows the knee to be maintained in position while the patient stands and then practises moving about in standing.

This man had problems with other components required for standing up, such as ankle dorsiflexion to bring his centre of gravity forward and knee extension throughout the action to enable weight to be taken through the affected leg. The necessary muscles will need to be trained, and the movement components practised in the appropriate part of the activity.

This man was able to *improve his performance* within a few minutes, but he will only *learn* to stand up and sit down correctly if he has the opportunity for consistent practice *(Step 4)*. The therapist will therefore ensure that the other relevant health professionals (particularly the nurse and occupational therapist) and relatives give him this opportunity. If he is allowed to practise

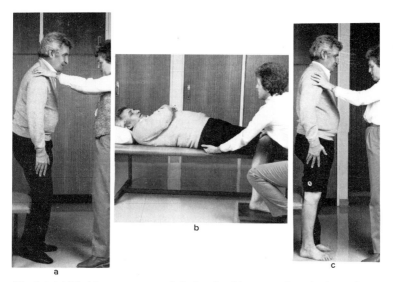

Fig. 3.2 (a) His hips are not extended; therefore his centre of gravity is too far back. (b) Training to improve hip extension in a position in which he need concentrate only on this component. (c) When he stands up again his lower limb alignment is improved.

incorrectly (for example, with all his weight taken through his intact leg), he will not be able to transfer what he has begun to learn in physiotherapy sessions into his everyday life. Inconsistency of practice will lead to confusion and interfere with the learning process. He may actually learn a method of standing up which is biomechanically inferior to the method he is practising with the therapist.

The above example illustrates how muscle activity is elicited and trained in the context for which it is required. This may be significant both for behavioural and physiological reasons. It is known that an adult learning a new motor skill, for example a new sport, practises the skill itself. A windsurfer practises by sailing his board on the water (Fig. 3.3). In learning a new skill, muscles must be trained to contract with appropriate force and timing, at the correct length, in conjunction with the other necessary muscles. For example, in a normal subject, the ability of the triceps brachii to contract for the requirements of push-ups on the floor, does not mean that the same subject can control the triceps sufficiently well to throw a dart into the centre of a dartboard. The triceps will have to be trained for this activity. Hence the subject will practise the

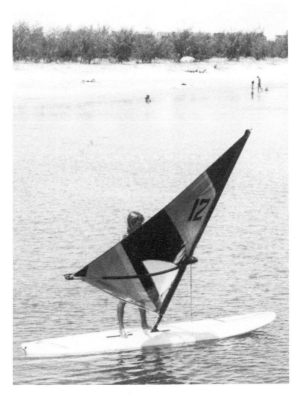

Fig. 3.3 The muscle action required for balancing of the sailboard and handling the sail is learned by practice of the activity itself.

activity itself until the triceps (and the other muscles involved) can perform to his satisfaction (so he wins the game). The length–tension relationship is considered a fundamental property of contracting muscle. Hence, for a stroke patient trying to elicit muscle activity and regain motor control, it may be that training of muscles within particular functional contexts enables the neuro-muscular system to re-establish appropriate length–tension relationships.

Balancing activities should also be trained in context. Balance is needed in everyday life under three conditions; most commonly, whenever we move in any non-supported position, but also when-ever the surface on which we sit or stand moves (on a boat or train), and whenever we are moved by someone else (when jostled in a crowd, playing contact games). The two therapeutic models for improving balance which are in current use separate balance from functional activity. The techniques are aimed either at stimulating 'automatic reactions' to shifts in the centre of gravity brought about by the therapist, or at training the patient to remain motionless.

In the MRP, emphasis in balance training initially is on the patient initiating motor activity and controlling it, rather than on responding to displacement by an outside force.

Example 3. Balanced sitting
This man (Fig. 3.4a) is having difficulty maintaining the sitting position. Whenever he moves his head or lifts his arm he falls towards the left side or backwards. The therapist encourages him to reach forwards toward the floor (Fig. 3.4b) and sit up again. She gives manual guidance and verbal feedback to correct his alignment as he moves. Manual guidance ensures that he will not fall but is not so marked as to make him feel 'secure'. In training balanced movement the patient needs to feel physically 'insecure' in order to make the appropriate motor adjustments. Emotional security is provided by the relationship between therapist and patient, in which the patient *knows* the therapist will not allow him to fall. He also practises reaching sideways and looking over his shoulder and up to the ceiling, under the same training conditions as above. The therapist needs to remind the patient to look at what he is doing as visual training is an important part of motor training.

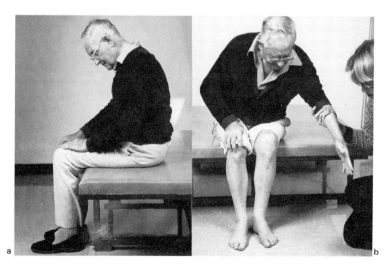

Fig. 3.4 (a) Although this man appears stable he was unable to move without falling backwards or to the side. (b) Part of training to improve his ability to move about in sitting.

In this example the patient is learning how to initiate movement himself and to control that movement. This method of training takes advantage of the fact that balance can only improve for a particular activity if that activity is practised. For example, balancing in sitting or standing involves being able to move about in these positions without losing control. Lawther (1977) cites several studies which indicate that balance is highly specific in terms of particular activities and positions.

Techniques

Certain techniques are probably crucial for eliciting muscle activity, and for motor learning to take place.

1. Manual guidance

Manual guidance is given by the therapist to ensure that limb and trunk alignment favours the muscle action required for the particular activity being trained. Manual guidance may include taking some of the weight of a limb or preventing a limb from persistently adopting a position which favours contraction of incorrect muscles.

> *Example 4. Upper limb function*
> This woman (Fig. 3.5a) is having difficulty eliciting activity in the wrist extensors when asked to extend the wrist and move the bottle back on the table. When the therapist holds her wrist and forearm in an alignment which favours extensor carpi radialis (Fig. 3.5b), active radial deviation is quickly elicited (Fig. 3.5c). She is then able to transfer this activity to extension of the wrist and move the bottle as requested.

In the above example, manual guidance ensured that the *alignment* favoured the muscles required to contract. If the wrist is held in a position in which extensor carpi radialis is lengthened in line with the pull of gravity, the effect of the weight of the hand and the lengthened state of the muscle may trigger off activity in that muscle.

Once some motor control has been established, excessive manual guidance will interfere with practice. When a patient can activate the necessary muscles and switch off unnecessary activity, it may be better for him to practise with verbal feedback or to practise alone following a set of instructions or guidelines. If the therapist holds his limb too firmly the patient does not have the chance to experiment and work out for himself what corrections are needed.

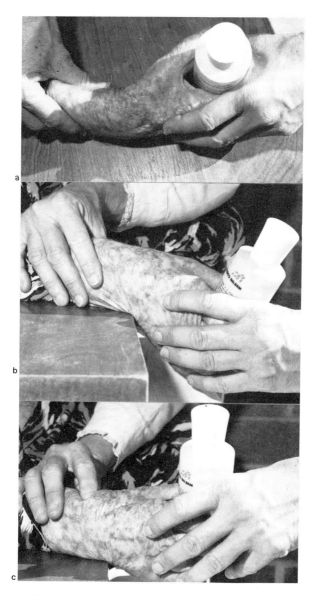

Fig. 3.5 (a) She is unable to activate her extensor carpi radialis in this position. (b) & (c) She can, however, activate her radial extensor in this position, and then transfer this muscle activity to wrist extension as required in 5(a).

Example 5. Upper limb function
This woman (Fig. 3.6) has some control over her shoulder muscles but insufficient to practise in sitting without substitution movements. Once the therapist has lifted her arm into the vertical position, the patient is able to practise moving her arm about and gradually increase the range over which she has control. The therapist gives verbal feedback about alignment but manual guidance is only intermittent and involves slight corrections if the patient is about to lose control. The therapist remains ready to take hold of or guide the arm but only if necessary.

It may be necessary initially to hold the entire limb, or to hold a segment of the limb in order to give sufficient stability to enable a muscle to contract.

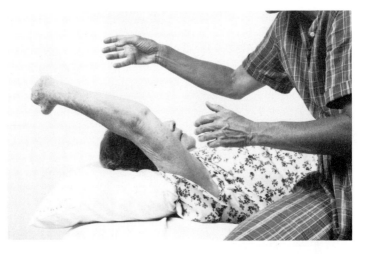

Fig. 3.6 Training to improve control over muscles around shoulder. She is practising controlling eccentric and concentric activity and changing from one type of activity to the other.

Example 6. Standing up and sitting down
This woman is having difficulty standing up (Fig. 3.7). She cannot keep her foot firmly on the floor and she is standing up with more weight on her intact left side. The therapist is using manual guidance to ensure the correct ankle-knee alignment and to hold the patient's right foot firmly on the floor. The downwards pressure and the guidance of the knee forward gives the stability which enables the patient to contract her anterior tibial muscles and helps her to take some weight through that foot. The patient thinks about pushing down through her right foot as she practises standing up.

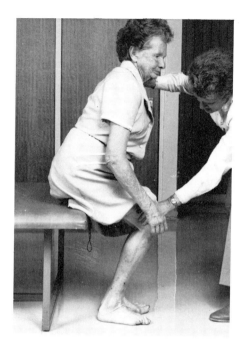

Fig. 3.7 Training to improve alignment of affected leg while standing up. This will provide the stability to enable the quadriceps and anterior tibial muscles to develop control while under a load.

The therapist, when giving manual guidance, should ensure that assistance or guidance results in the patient actually contracting a muscle and doing part of the activity. Otherwise therapy becomes a passive intervention with the therapist lifting the patient or passively moving a limb. In addition, too firm a hold on a limb may prevent the therapist from sensing a weak muscle contraction and giving this feedback to the patient.

2. Feedback, instruction, explanation

In terms of movement, feedback gives knowledge of motor performance (KP) and knowledge of the results (KR) of that performance. Feedback, together with *explanation* and clear *instruction*, enables the patient to participate with the therapist in working out solutions to his motor problems. The feedback techniques used in training are principally auditory (verbal) and visual.

The therapist gives *verbal feedback* throughout the training process to monitor the patient's performance and give him information as to whether or not his performance is correct, at what point the movement goes wrong or at what point inappropriate muscle activity is interfering with the movement.

Verbal feedback is used carefully as a reinforcer. Only a successful performance, not merely a good try, is rewarded by 'good', 'yes, that's right', so the patient knows exactly what he must repeat.

Fitts (1964) proposed three stages in learning a motor skill, cognitive, associative and autonomous. As with motor skill learning in the non brain-damaged, the early stage of learning or relearning following stroke is cognitive and requires verbal cues, explanations and instructions which help the patient think things through. Where a patient is having difficulty understanding language, verbal information is augmented or replaced by non-verbal means of communication, such as gesture, demonstration and video recording.

Clear identification of the goal to be pursued, both long and short term, helps the cognitive process, but probably only if the goal is relevant and worthwhile for what the patient perceives as his needs. Practice sessions which simulate everyday situations makes the adjustment from therapy session to everyday life relatively easy.

Example 7. Upper limb function
A patient who is having difficulty abducting his thumb, may be better able to elicit activity in abductor pollicis brevis if he is asked to take hold of a glass (which requires abduction at the carpo-meta-carpal joint) than if he is asked to move his thumb away from his hand.

The patient is encouraged to use *visual feedback* not only for KP and KR but to provide spatial cues. In order to move about (alter our position in space) we need both internal and external feedback. Until recently, visual receptors have been considered to be of relatively minor importance in balanced movement, receptors in vestibular and musculo-skeletal systems being thought more important (Gydikov et al, 1973; Stein et al, 1973). However, recent studies have shown that vision has a proprioceptive role in maintaining a balanced alignment as we move about.

Lee and Lishman (1975), from their experiments with adults, concluded that 'visual proprioceptive information is generally more sensitive than mechanical proprioceptive information from the vestibular system and the ankles and feet . . .'. De Wit (1972) showed that a person's standing balance could be experimentally controlled by manipulating his visual information. De Wit's subjects swayed laterally in phase with a moving rod. Lee and Aronson (1974) studied toddlers standing in an experimental room of movable walls and ceiling. The toddlers corrected their standing position according to their visual information, swaying with the room often to the extent of falling over.

Deficient visual perception may be a significant factor in the poor balance seen in some stroke patients, particularly those who are older. Several authors (Bruell et al, 1954; Birch et al, 1962; de Cencio et al, 1970) have shown that perception of verticality in the stroke patients they studied deviated significantly from normal. Tobis and associates (1981) studied 134 elderly subjects with a history of falls and found that the fallers made significant errors in the visual perception of the verticality or horizontality of a rod.

Analysis of verticality and horizontality perception should be performed on any stroke patient who is having difficulty moving about in standing, and a training programme should be designed specifically for this problem.

A demonstration by the therapist will provide visual feedback of the discrepancies between the patient's and the normal performance of an activity. Instantaneous visual feedback from watching his own performance on a T.V. monitor will enable him to compare his performance as he senses it internally with what he sees on a videotape.

Example 8. Standing balance
A man who had had little therapy since his stroke several months earlier was unable to stand alone. He fell towards one side or the other, backward or forward. He did not improve when given practice of reaching out with his hand or looking over his shoulder, or when an attempt was made to train postural sway by alternate displacements of his centre of gravity produced by the therapist. He stated that he sensed he was falling only when he was already seen to have swayed a considerable distance from the mid position. As he appeared to be receiving delayed information about his alignment, he was provided on a video monitor with immediate visual information about his position. He watched the monitor as he attempted to stand alone. He was able to correct his excessive body sway by adjusting his alignment according to the errors he saw. During his first practice session, he stood for two minutes without assistance.

3. Part-whole practice

The relative effectiveness of practising the whole activity, or practising part of the activity followed by the whole activity, has been studied in non brain-damaged subjects. Following stroke, it is usually necessary for a patient to practise first the muscle activity required for a particular movement component with which he is having difficulty, and this practice is then followed by practice of the whole activity with particular attention to the difficult component.

However, there are also times when it may be necessary for the patient to practise the whole activity, even though he needs a great deal of assistance from the therapist. It may be that this gives him the idea of the rhythm, timing and speed of the activity as well as of the temporal and spatial sequencing of the components.

4. Muscle training

In the training of motor control following stroke, certain factors about the structure and function of muscle should be considered:

Classes of muscle contraction. In normal activities, muscles are required to perform shortening (concentric) contractions, lengthening (eccentric) contractions and to contract without changing length (isometric).

Activity can frequently be elicited in an apparently inactive muscle if it is encouraged to *contract while lengthening*. Once activity is elicited in this way, a shortening contraction can usually be performed. This occurs because elastic (mechanical) energy is stored in the series elastic elements as the muscle is stretched, and the muscle then needs to generate less energy when it contracts to shorten. When a shortening contraction is attempted first, energy must come from the chemical energy generated by the contractile component of the muscle (Cavagna, 1968; Cavagna et al 1971) and this may be impossible if the patient is having difficulty eliciting any motor control.

> *Example 9. Upper limb function*
> This woman (Fig. 3.8) was not able to extend her elbow. However, when asked to lower her hand gently to her head, without letting her hand drop, she was able to activate her triceps brachii through part of middle range. When she could control this eccentric contraction of her triceps to some extent, she was able to extend her elbow through part of range. The eliciting of a lengthening contraction was the first step in gaining control of elbow extension. Now she practises moving her elbow through full range, controlling the muscle activity as she shifts from a concentric to an eccentric contraction.

One of the advantages of training within specific functional contexts is that the patient practises making the necessary changes in the

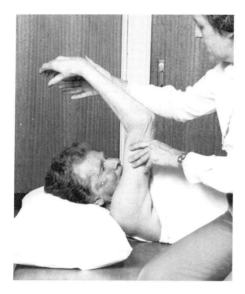

Fig. 3.8 Training to improve control over the triceps. In progressing the activity, the therapist will give less assistance to the shoulder so the shoulder position will also have to be controlled.

muscle work required normally for the activity. For example, changes from a shortening contraction of one group of muscles to a lengthening contraction in the antagonist group as occurs when the arm is raised above the head in supine; changes from a shortening contraction in one group to a lengthening contraction in the same group as occurs when the arm is lifted above the head then lowered in the sitting position.

Energy expenditure. A muscle may not be able to contract to move a limb in a controlled manner if that muscle is required to expend more energy than it can generate.

> *Example 10. Upper limb function*
> This woman (Fig. 3.9a) is not able to flex her arm forward or abduct it without substituting shoulder girdle elevation for the last few degrees of movement. That is, her deltoid is not well enough controlled to raise the weight of the arm. She can, however, flex and abduct the shoulder without substitution strategies in a position in which the weight of the limb is less and if the angle of pull of the deltoid muscle involves less gravity resistance (Figs. 3.9b & 3.9c). She can practise these movements on her own, with her arm resting on a table at right-angles to her body.

Muscle length. Both in eliciting activity in apparently inactive muscle and in training control for specific functions, the length at

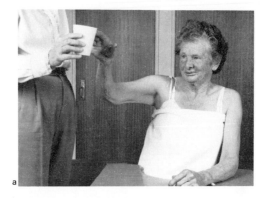

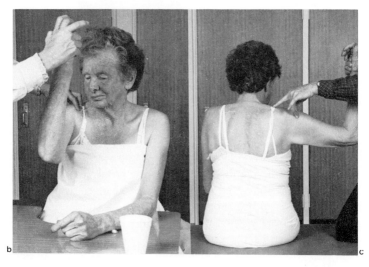

Fig. 3.9 (a) Note the incorrect relationship between humeral and scapular movement. There is insufficient control of the deltoid at this length and in this relationship to gravity. (b) Training to improve control of the deltoid in this position. The therapist is taking some of the weight of the arm, but will gradually decrease this assistance. (c) Training of the deltoid as abductor in the movement range at which control is poor. Again the therapist assists by taking some of the weight of the limb.

which the muscle is required to contract for each specific function appears a significant point to consider. Gossman and associates (1982), in discussing the results of animal experiments, suggest that emphasis in muscle training should be on 'restoring normal length and developing tension at the appropriate point in the range'.

Elimination of unnecessary muscle activity. Efficient movement may be described as the successful performance of an activity, utilising minimum amounts of muscular tension. It involves the ability to localise appropriate muscle activity according to the task being performed (Rosenbloom & Horton, 1971). The literature contains many studies on normal subjects which stress the importance of the inhibition of unnecessary activity in the learning of motor control and skill in sporting activities, novel motor tasks and during motor development in children. Broer and Zernicke (1979) comment that muscular control is the ability to prevent from contracting those muscles which do not contribute to the maintenance of the position or the execution of the movement. MacConaill and Basmajian (1969) point out that expenditure of energy should be the minimum necessary to allow the desired activity to be achieved.

Example 11. Oro-motor function
This man (Fig. 3.10a), five days after his stroke, has poor muscular control of the lower third of his face. He also has overactivity of his intact R. side and these two factors make it difficult for him to open his mouth symmetrically and close his jaw with even lip closure. His facial expressions are asymmetrical. These problems are explained to him and he is instructed to relax the muscles on the intact side of his face (Fig. 3.10b) while he practises opening his mouth. The therapist monitors the patient's performance verbally and as soon as he is able to eliminate the overactivity on the intact side of his face he is able to elicit activity in the appropriate muscles on the affected side of his face (Fig. 3.10c).

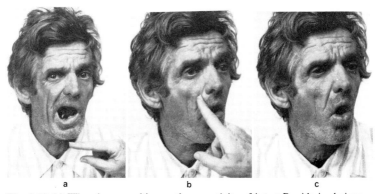

a   b   c

Fig. 3.10 (a) When he opens his mouth overactivity of intact R. side is obvious. There is little activity on the L. side. (b) Training to decrease activity of the intact side. (c) When he opens his mouth a few minutes later, in order that the therapist can re-evaluate his performance, he shows some improvement.

Whether the stroke patient learns to activate the correct muscles, with correct tension and force, in the correct range, and therefore move efficiently with an appropriate amount of energy expenditure, will depend to some extent on the training he receives.

It is probable that some therapeutic techniques in current use, such as the stimulation of mass movement patterns, resistive techniques which allow or encourage overflow into other muscle groups and encouragement of movement of the intact side to assist the affected side, prevent the patient from learning to activate muscles selectively and to cease muscle activity once initiated. The patient may actually be prevented from re-establishing the best possible motor control. In other words, practice which involves either (a) contracting the wrong muscle/s for a particular movement or activity (that is, substituting a 'strong' muscle for a 'weak' muscle) or (b) overflow of activity into muscles not necessary for performance of the task either on the intact or affected side, probably interferes with the regaining of motor control.

In the MRP, muscle activity is trained as a general principle within specific functional contexts. In oro-motor function, when activity of the tongue is difficult to elicit, it may be necessary to stimulate the tongue directly in order to improve swallowing.

Example 12. Oro-motor function
The man in Figure 3.10 was also having difficulty swallowing because his tongue was flaccid, too far forward in his mouth and was not able to assume the shapes necessary for swallowing. Digital stimulation to his tongue (Fig. 3.11a) combined with training of jaw closure with lips evenly together (Fig. 3.11b), result in improved swallowing.

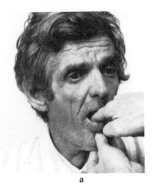 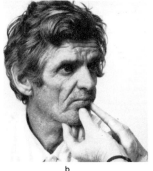

a   b

Fig. 3.11 (a) Digital stimulation in a lateral direction to the tongue, immediately followed by: (b) Training of lip and jaw closure with swallowing.

Oro-motor problems are very distressing both for the patient and his relatives, who find his dribbling and difficulty controlling food embarrassing. These problems respond very quickly to early intervention, prevent the use of a nasogastric tube, improve the patient's self-esteem and enable him to enjoy his meals again and feel comfortable and ready to socialise during meal times. Improved control prevents wiping of the mouth from becoming an habitual response which interferes with the patient's ability to concentrate and participate in his training programme.

RATIONALE FOR EARLY MOTOR TRAINING

That active rehabilitation should start immediately the patient's vital signs are stable is a widespread belief. However, the reasons for this are rarely clearly defined. The presence of differing opinions about the type of early rehabilitation may be an indication that the objectives of rehabilitation do not always reflect the current state of knowledge in various relevant areas. The rationale for early motor training can be based on the results of both physiological and behavioural studies. The aims of early training can be expressed in terms of the need:

1. To take advantage of the *learning capacity* and *adaptability of the brain*; that is, to ensure that the patient learns the appropriate motor functions rather than compensatory or substitution movements.
2. To prevent
    (a) *disabling muscle imbalance* which results from soft tissue tightness, muscle overactivity, and incorrect motor learning;
    (b) *learned non-use* of the affected limbs;
    (c) *soft tissue injury*;
    (d) *disuse effects* (such as muscle atrophy, bone demineralisation, decreased cardio-pulmonary function).

In addition, early training in standing seems to overcome urinary incontinence which otherwise requires catheterization. Early training of oro-motor control improves swallowing which overcomes the tendency to dribble saliva. Early gains in these two areas of function cause a marked improvement in the patient's self-esteem and in the motivation which is necessary if rehabilitation is to be successful.

A review of the preventative aspects of early training raises interesting points for future investigation.

(a) Muscle imbalance

The patient immediately following his stroke demonstrates depressed motor function with an inability to move, that is to activate muscles on the affected side. There is a disruption of selective neurocontrol. Gradually there is some return of muscle activity.

From the moment the patient attempts to move, there is a tendency for muscle imbalance to develop. As he tries hard to accomplish the desired activity he has a tendency to make several types of error:

1. He may activate the incorrect muscles for a particular activity. For example, if he tries to flex his shoulder with an absent or insufficient contraction of his shoulder flexors, he may substitute excessive shoulder girdle elevation for shoulder flexion.
2. He may move the intact side instead of the affected side. For example, in standing, when the therapist instructs him to straighten his knee, he may only activate the quadriceps on the intact side; he may clench his fist on his intact side as he tries to lift his affected arm.
3. He may demonstrate abnormal synergic muscle activity. Once this becomes habitual (learned), certain muscles will always contract together. For example, when he holds an object, he may use his wrist and elbow flexors at the same time as his finger flexors.
4. He may be able to contract a muscle but not sustain the contraction for the necessary time. For example, he may be able to contract his quadriceps and straighten his knee briefly in standing but may not be able to sustain the contraction.
5. He may contract a muscle too strongly for the needs of the movement, that is, activate too many motor units. For example, when he picks up a polystyrene cup he will hold it too firmly and deform it.

In addition, the patient, because it is difficult to move, tends to remain in the same position for long periods (Fig. 3.12), with muscles persistently held in either a shortened or lengthened position. This will cause changes within the muscles themselves and these changes will start to occur within a short time. It is a common observation that tissue flexibility decreases progressively as the period of inactivity lengthens (Perry, 1980). Gossman and associates (1982) report animal studies which have shown that 'when muscle is subjected to imposed maintained changes in length, it undergoes

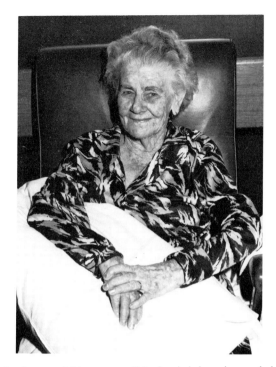

Fig. 3.12 Persistence of this posture will lead to imbalance in muscle length.

anatomical, biochemical and physiological changes that are not immediately obvious nor readily considered'. These 'length-associated changes can be induced by immobilisation . . . muscle imbalance, postural malalignment . . .'. They go on to point out that the changes within muscle are more pronounced when the muscle is shortened than when it is lengthened.

In the stroke patient, it may be that movement errors plus the length-associated changes in muscle caused by persistence of position over a period of time will together result in more disability than that caused by the original brain damage.

Gossman and associates (1982) point out that a muscle which has shortened may appear 'strong' if it is tested in its optimal adapted position, whereas a muscle which is lengthened may appear 'weak' because the evaluation is not performed at its optimal test length. They suggest that the associated changes in the passive tension of the shortened muscle through shortening of the connective tissue elements contributes to the clinically perceived 'strength' of the muscle. For various reasons, such as position, certain muscles will tend to shorten. These muscles will tend to contract spontaneously (such as during a cough) and if they are also shortened in length there may be a greater tendency both for them to contract spontaneously and for them to contract instead of the required, but lengthened, muscles whenever the patient tries to move. It is observable clinically that the patient tries to hasten recovery by practising whatever movement he can perform. If this is so, over-activity in shortened muscle would be a major factor contributing to increasing muscle imbalance and would give the appearance of what is called 'spasticity'. It is probable that the so-called 'spasticity' described following stroke has a muscular component (short-ened muscle tending to contract strongly) as well as a neural component (hyperactive motoneuron pool). That is, 'spasticity' may really be a combination of muscle tightness and muscle overactivity.

In addition, movement errors become habitual, that is, well learned. Perry (1980) has suggested a link between muscle short-ening and spasticity, commenting that while there are 'no controlled studies indicating that prevention of contracture reduces spasticity, many experiences support this concept'. The authors' clinical experience with early training of muscle activity as part of the MRP indicates that while poor motor control is a problem following stroke most patients do not develop obvious signs of spasticity.

The re-emergence of muscle activity in individual muscles is therefore a crucial event in terms of the patient's eventual recovery of function. Whether the patient develops muscle tightness and muscle overactivity may depend upon the type of therapy he receives. At this time, the therapist should be training the patient to activate and gain control over specific muscles for a particular activity, correcting trunk and limb alignment, maintaining the normal resting length of muscles, in particular ensuring that muscles which rest in their shortened position do not become tight. Motor training requires the therapist to recognise any unnecessary tension in muscles not involved in the activity being trained, as well as either excessive or unsustained activity in the muscles which are being trained. The patient must be guided to contract muscles appropriately, for example, eliminate unnecessary muscle tension or sustain a contraction at a particular point of that muscle's length.

(b) Learned non use

The patient who is left to struggle on his own or who is encouraged or allowed to use his intact limbs to compensate for lack of movement of his affected side may learn not to use the affected limbs. Taub (1980), as a result of many experiments with monkeys, proposed that the lack of purposive movement in a unilaterally deafferented upper limb is due primarily to a learning phenomenon which he has called 'learned non-use'. Various experiments have shown that monkeys do not use the affected upper limb when only this limb has been deafferented, whereas, when bilateral deafferentation is carried out, the motor deficit is far less, with movement which approximates the normal being exhibited.

Taub's studies have shown that when a monkey with a single limb deafferented has the intact limb restrained, he will use the affected limb. If training of the affected limb is added to restraint of the intact limb, he will regain useful function of the affected limb.

Taub suggests that learned non-use may be related to motivation. The monkey with an unrestrained intact limb can use this to satisfy most of his wants. He has discovered, immediately following surgery, that he cannot use his affected limb and he therefore learns *not* to use it; that is, the habit persists. When the limb becomes potentially useful, the habit of non-use is so persistent that the monkey does not *know* that he *could* use the limb. Motivation to use this limb no longer exists.

As Taub hypothesises, learned non-use may also be a factor in the relative non-recovery of upper limb function in people following stroke (Taub, 1980). For a period following the stroke, it can be difficult to elicit activity in the affected upper limb. Although limited muscle activity is usually present under certain conditions, when the patient tries to perform everyday functions muscle activity is not sufficient for these functions to be carried out. However, much of what the patient wants to do at this stage can be accomplished with the intact limb. If, in addition, all attempts to move the affected limb fail repeatedly, motivation to use the limb will decrease. The patient learns *not* to use the limb. According to Taub, lack of motor activity may be due more to lack of motivation and a learned helplessness than to a basic motor incapacity.

The experience of the authors is that (i) a *demonstration* to the patient in the early stages following his stroke that he has some muscle activity in his upper limb, (ii) an *explanation* that he will be tempted to substitute his intact limb for the affected limbs, (iii) *instructions* to cut down activity in the intact limb to the minimum necessary during the day and to eliminate it completely in training sessions, and (iv) a *training programme* which is begun immediately and is directed at eliciting specific muscle activity and increasing motor control (Carr & Shepherd, 1982) result in better recovery of function than is generally reported in the literature. It appears from the studies which have so far been done (Schwartzman, 1974; Ostendorf & Wolf, 1981) that periods of restraint of the intact limb will further increase the capacity of patients to regain effective function.

(c) Soft tissue injury

Soft tissue injury with pain and stiffness can develop in the presence of depressed motor function through incorrect handling of paretic limbs of anyone who comes in contact with the patient or by the patient himself. Soft tissue injury is particularly common to the gleno-humeral joint (GHJ) and its surroundings. The patient will respond to pain by holding his limb stiffly and by developing substitution movements which will further aggravate muscle imbalance.

Loose capsule and ligaments render the GHJ intrinsically weak (Nepomuceno & Miller, 1974). Therefore, if soft tissues are allowed to elongate in the early stage following stroke while muscles are relatively inactive, it is possible that this 'joint weakness'may itself interfere with the gaining of muscular control of the shoulder.

In the absence of muscle support and protection, soft tissue injury may be brought about by several factors, occurring either in isolation or in combination:

(i) Handling of a joint unprotected by normal muscle constitutes a potential strain and should be carried out with care and due regard to normal alignment and joint relationships. Forced passive range of movement should be avoided. This includes self-ranging exercises of the GHJ.

Pulling on the relatively unprotected shoulder in order to help the patient sit up or stand may also stretch or tear the soft tissues around the shoulder. Frequent passive range of motion exercises or pulling on the arm may result in repetition injury, an inflammatory process which, without appropriate intervention, will result in chronic pain and stiffness due to a thickening of capsule and ligaments.

Passive range of motion exercises, because they cannot be controlled by the inactive muscles surrounding the joint, may force an abnormal relationship between humerus and scapula because passive movement of the GHJ will not necessarily be combined with the corresponding and necessary movement of the scapula. The overall relationship between gleno-humeral and scapulo-thoracic movement during abduction is normally about 2:1. In the first 30 of abduction the ratio is 4:1 but this becomes 5:4 beyond this point (Poppen & Walker, 1976). Without this concomittent movement the head of the humerus will impinge on the acromion process. In addition, forced abduction of the GHJ without external rotation impinges the tuberosity cuff ligament zone on to the acromion process which may result in rupture of the rotator cuff. Flexion and abduction of the GHJ create friction–compression stress between the humeral head and coracoacromial ligament.

(ii) The integrity of the shoulder joint depends to a large extent on muscular support. The effect of limb weight in the upright position combined with immobility of the arm is a gradual displacement downward of the head of the humerus due to distension of the joint capule, with stretching of the muscles and ligaments leading to *subluxation*. Subluxation is, therefore, commonly found in patients who spend long periods in a position which allows the GHJ to become distracted. When the shoulder is moved passively the stretched capsule may become nipped between the joint surfaces causing pain. Subluxation appears, therefore, to be associated with shoulder pain despite comments to the contrary by some authors.

The decision to use slings in the prevention of subluxation and/or pain of the GHJ is controversial as is the type of sling to use. There are no definitive studies. However, it appears obvious that the unprotected shoulder needs support when the patient is standing and walking. The Hook hemi-harness* is probably the most satisfactory sling under these circumstances if it is correctly applied. The most important factor in maintaining joint integrity, however, is the retraining of muscle activity around the shoulder in order that the muscles themselves can re-establish their usual supporting function.

(iii) Many elderly patients may be predisposed to a painful shoulder because of pre-existing shoulder 'stiffness', muscle tightness, or joint pathology (Caillet, 1980). Degenerative changes are known to develop in the rotator cuff with increasing age (Moseley, 1963).

* Created by the Orthopedic Equipment Company, Bourbon, Indiana, U.S.A. 46504, in conjunction with the August E. Hook Physical Rehabilitation Center.

Prevention of soft tissue stretching, tightness and injury is probably essential if the patient is to gain motor control and participate fully in his training programme. Any complaint of pain should be analysed to establish a cause so that the necessary therapy can be commenced. Unfortunately, without an analysis of the cause of pain, the therapist may react to a complaint of pain and stiffness by increasing passive range of motion exercises in the belief that inactivity is causing the pain. This will cause further trauma and an increase of symptoms. Any patient who has a demonstrable musculo-skeletal lesion of the shoulder region requires a similar intervention (for example, peripheral joint mobilisation) for these problems as would be given to the non-stroke patient with shoulder problems.

(d) Disuse effects

The results of disuse of the neuromuscular system occur fairly rapidly, particularly in the elderly person. The stroke patient commonly spends a large part of his day in relative immobility.

Muscle has considerable capacity for accommodating to changes in demand, acquiring physiological and biochemical characteristics which are better suited to the new requirements. Immobilisation causes a decrease in metabolic demand (Salmons & Henriksson, 1981).

Disuse changes include muscle atrophy due to a decrease in number and size of muscle fibres, muscle tightness, demineralisation of bone, and changes in the cardio-pulmonary system resulting in decreased oxygen delivery. These changes will result in a decrease in muscle strength, endurance and flexibility throughout the body and not just in the affected limbs. Disuse also appears to affect mental functioning, causing a generalised debility and lethargy.

Many stroke patients are elderly and many have been relatively inactive before their stroke. These are still no guidelines as to whether the physiological changes seen in the elderly person are due to age or to an inactive life style (Payton, 1983). Nevertheless, many stroke patients probably present post-stroke with pre-existing disuse effects and these will be increased by the immobility which results from depressed motor function and institutionalisation. For example, an elderly person having difficulty standing up and sitting down may have had difficulty before his stroke because of weak quadriceps muscles. Prolonged sitting (that is, disuse) after the stroke will increase muscle weakness and cause some shortening of the hamstrings which will make it increasingly difficult to activate the quadriceps in their shortened position.

Therapy sessions which include training of standing up and sitting down, stepping forward with the intact leg in standing and practice of moving about in standing, will, in addition to improving motor control, prevent disuse effects and increase the person's endurance.

THE ENVIRONMENT

It is probable that some of the failure of modern rehabilitation for stroke is the result of the impoverished non-challenging environment in which many patients find themselves.

Rehabilitation should commence as soon as the patient's vital signs are stable and the patient should be introduced quickly to normal activities and interests. Mental ability is necessary for effective motor retraining and there is evidence that mental health is promoted by encouragement to lead a relatively normal daily life (Robinson, 1976). Studies of time-use by stroke patients in three rehabilitation settings (Keith, 1980; Keith & Sharpe, 1980) indicate that stroke patients spend more time in passive solitary behaviour than in therapeutic activities.

One outcome of a poor environment may be a mental deterioration which is unrelated to pre-stroke mental condition or age but due instead to inactivity, depression and disuse of mental faculties (Walsh & Greenough, 1976). The patient should get up and dressed. His day should take on a relatively normal routine, with times set aside for recreation, mental and motor training programmes and socialisation, as well as any other specific therapy programmes, such as speech therapy, which may be needed.

It is recognised that the patient who is unmotivated will not succeed in rehabilitation (Nicholas, 1980). However, lack of motivation needs to be analysed with each particular patient in order to find a solution. In rehabilitation centres and stroke units motivation needs to be organised rather than left to chance, and the environment should be planned in order to motivate the patient towards recovery (Carr & Shepherd, 1982). There is evidence from animal studies that an enriched environment plays a significant part in recovery from brain damage (Rosenzweig et al, 1967; Walsh & Greenough, 1975; Walsh, 1981) and the brain changes seen to develop are probably due to the increased opportunities for learning which are present in an environment which is rich, varied and challenging.

Clinical observations indicate that success early in the retraining process has a significant motivating effect, particularly if the success is experienced in some activity relevant to the patient's hopes for the future. Early success in the accomplishment of sitting and standing, that is, the ability to move about in these positions, and in gaining small amounts of muscle activity in the upper limb, indicate to the patient that he is capable of working towards surmounting some of the obstacles which separate him from normal life. The provision of charts, videorecordings or a diary which demonstrate progress are also powerful motivators.

Therapy or training designed to improve motor function will only be effective if consistency of practice is organised. Although, when with the physiotherapist the patient's motor performance will improve, this correct performance will only be learned if there is opportunity to practise correctly during the time when the patient is not with the therapist. *Consistency of practice* needs to be organised. The patient needs to know what to practice and should be able to monitor his practice helped by a relative. Activities such as standing up and sitting down should be practised correctly each time the opportunity occurs.

In this chapter, a. motor control-motor learning paradigm is described as the basis upon which to build physiotherapy practice. This model depends upon skill in problem recognition and analysis, and this skill depends upon an understanding of the biomechanics, muscle biology, and behavioural and neural mechanisms which make up motor control and motor learning.

REFERENCES

Bennett E L 1976 Cerebral effects of differential experience and training. In: Rosenzweig M R, Bennett E L (eds) Neural mechanisms of learning and memory. The MIT Press, Cambridge, p 279–288

Birch H G, Belmont I, Reilly T, Belmont L 1962 Somesthetic influences in perception of visual verticality in hemiplegia. Archives of Physical Medicine and Rehabilitation 43: 556–560

Broer M R, Zernicke R F 1979 Efficiency of human movement, 4th edn. Saunders, Philadelphia

Bruell J H, Peczaczynski M, Volk D 1957 Disturbance of perception of verticality in patients with hemiplegia: second report. Archives of Physical Medicine and Rehabilitation 38: 776–780

Caillet R 1980 The shoulder in hemiplegia. F A Davis, Philadelphia

Carr J H, Shepherd R B 1982 A motor relearning programme for stroke. Heinemann, London

Cavagna G A, Dusman B, Margaria R 1968 Positive work done by a previously stretched muscle. Journal of Applied Physiology 24: 21–32

Cavagna G A, Komarek L, Citterio G, Margaria R 1971 Power output of the previously stretched muscle. Medicine and Sport 6. Karger, Basel.

de Cencio D V, Ledhner M, Voron D 1970 Verticality perception and ambulation in hemiplegia. Archives of Physical Medicine and Rehabilitation 51: 105–110

De Wit G 1972 Optic versus vestibular and proprioceptive impulses measured by posturometry. Agressologie 13B: 75–79

Dubois E 1960 Adult education and andgrogy. In: Spencer M, Door C (eds) Understanding aging: a multidisciplinary approach. Appleton Century Crofts, New York

Fitts P M 1964 Perceptual motor skill learning. In: Melton A W (ed) Categories of human learning. Academic Press, New York

Gibbs J R 1960 Learning theory and education. In: Knowles M K (ed) Handbook of adult education. Adult Education Association of USA, Chicago

Goldberger M 1980 Motor recovery after lesions. Trends in Neuroscience 3: 288–91

Gossman M R, Sahrmann S A, Ross S J 1982 Review of length-associated changes in muscle. Physical Therapy 62, 12: 1799–1808

Greenough W T 1980 Development and memory: the synaptic connection. In: Teyler T (ed) Brain and learning. Reidel Pub Co, Dordrecht, Holland

Gydikov A A, Tankov N T, Kosarov D S (eds) 1973 Motor control. Plenum Press, New York

Halberstam J L, Zaretsky H H 1969 Learning capacities of the elderly and brain damaged. Archives of Physical Medicine and Rehabilitation: 133–139

Inman V T, Ralston H J, Todd F 1981 Human walking. Williams & Wilkins, Baltimore

Keith R A 1980 Activity patterns of a stroke rehabilitation unit. Social Science and Medicine 14A: 575–580

Keith R A, Sharp K W 1980 Time use of stroke patients in three rehabilitation hospitals. Archives of physical Medicine and Rehabilitation 61: 501–503

Lawther J D 1977 The learning and performance of physical skills, 2nd edn. Prentice Hall, Englewood Cliffs, New Jersey

Lee D N, Aronson E 1974 Visual proprioceptive control of standing in human infants. Perception and Psychophysics 15: 529–532

Lee D N, Lishman J R 1975 Visual proprioceptive control of stance. Journal of Human Movement Studies 1: 87–95

Lynch G, Wells J 1980 Neuroanatomical plasticity and behavioural adaptabilty. In: Teyler T (ed) Brain and learning. Reidel Pub Co, Dordrecht, Holland

MacConaill M A, Basmajian J V 1969 Muscles and movements. Basis for human kinesiology. Williams & Wilkins, Baltimore

Moseley H F 1963 The vascular supply of the rotator cuff. Surgical Clinics of North America 43: 1521–1522

Nepomuceno C S, Miller J M 1974 Shoulder arthrography in hemiplegic patients. Archives of Physical Medicine and Rehabilitation 55: 49–51

Ostendorf C G, Wolf S L 1981 Effect of forced use of the upper extremity of a hemiplegic patient on changes in function. Physical Therapy 61: 1022–1028

Payton O 1983 Aging process. Implications for clinical practice. Physical Therapy 63, 1: 41–48

Perry J 1980 Rehabilitation of spasticity. In: Feldman R D (ed) Spasticity disorders of motor control. Symposia Specialist Inc, Chicago

Poppen N K, Walker P S 1976 Normal and abnormal motion of the shoulder. Journal of Bone and Joint Surgery 58A, 2: 195–201

Rasch P J, Morehouse C E 1957 Effect or static and dynamic exercises on muscular strength and hypertrophy. Journal of Applied Physiology 11: 29–34

Robinson R A 1976 Psychiatric aspects of stroke. In: Gillingham G, Mawdsley C, Williams A E (eds) Stroke. Churchill Livingstone, London

Rosenbloom L, Horton M E 1971 The maturation of fine prehension in young children. Developmental Medicine and Child Neurology 13: –8

Rosenzweig M R 1980 Responsiveness of brain size to individual experience: behavioural and evolutionary implications. In: Haln M, Jensen C, Dudek B (eds) Development and evaluation of brain size: behavioural implications. Academic Press, New York

Rosenzweig M R, Bennett E L, Diamond M C 1967 Effects of differential environment on brain anatomy and brain chemistry. Proceedings of the American Psychopathological Association 56: 45–46

Sale D, MacDougal D 1981 Specificity in strength training: a review for the coach and athlete. Canadian Journal of Applied Sport Sciences 6.2: 87–92

Salmons S, Henriksson J 1981 The adaptive response of skeletal muscle to increased use. Muscle and Nerve 4: 94–105

Saunders J B, Inman V T, Eberhart H D 1953 The major determinants in normal and pathological gait. Journal of Bone and Joint Surgery 35A; 3: 543–548

Schwartzman R J 1974 Rehabilitation of infantile hemiplegia. American Journal of Physical Medicine 53, 2: 75–81

Stein R B, Pearson K G, Smith R S, Redford J B (eds) 1973 Control of posture and locomotion. Plenum Press, New York

Taub E 1980 Somato-sensory deafferentation research with monkeys: implications for rehabilitation medicine. In: Ince L P (ed) Behavioural psychology in rehabilitation medicine: clinical applications. Williams & Wilkins, Baltimore

Tobis J S, Nayak L, Hochler F 1981 Visual perception of verticality and horizontality among elderly fallers. Archives of Physical Medicine and Rehabilitation 62: 619–622

Travis A M, Woolsey C W 1952 Motor abilities of adult macaca macatta following bilateral precentral and supplementary area lesions. Abstracted American Journal of Physiology 171–774

Travis A M, Woolsey C W 1956 Motor performance of monkeys after bilateral, partial and total cerebral decortications. American Journal of Physical Medicine 35: 273–310

Walsh R N 1981 Sensory environments, brain damage and drugs: a review of interactions and mediating mechanism. International Journal of Neuroscience 14: 129–137

Walsh R N, Cummins R A 1976 Neural responses to therapeutic environments. In: Walsh R N, Greenough W (eds) Environments as therapy for brain dysfunction. Plenum Press, New York

Walsh R, Greenough W (eds) 1976 Environments as therapy for brain dysfunction. Plenum Press, New York

Whiting H T A 1980 Dimensions of control in motor learning. In: Stelmark G E, Requin J (eds) Tutorials in motor behaviour. North Holland Pub Co, Amsterdam

Winter D A 1979 Biomechanics of human movement. John Wiley, New York

Recent findings on the neural control of locomotion: implications for the rehabilitation of gait

In the retraining of a patient's functional locomotor ability following stroke, rehabilitation techniques aim to achieve a normal gait pattern. This involves attempts to retrain normal patterns of muscle activity and joint excursion in the affected leg and should result in the most efficient and also the most aesthetically pleasing gait. However, there are many conflicting methods used to try and achieve this aim (see Bobath, 1980; Brunnström, 1970; Perry, 1980). It is fundamental that patients should receive the treatment that is most effective, and therefore attempts must be made to evaluate which techniques are most relevant physiologically. This can best be achieved by identifying the physiological parameters concerned with the initiation and modification of gait and then studying their alteration following stroke. Recent findings concerning the neural control of locomotion give an indication of some important parameters and these have also been observed to be altered following stroke. They should provide useful criteria for use in the retraining of gait following stroke, for the evaluation of recovery of normal gait, and as the basis for comparing the different methods used for gait retraining.

This chapter forms a review of some of the recently published literature concerning the neural control of locomotion and the neurophysiology of spasticity. It concentrates particularly on the attempts to identify some of the physiological parameters concerned with the initiation and modification of gait.

It concludes with suggestions on further studies which need to be made and also with suggestions on the most relevant approaches to gait retraining following stroke, as indicated at the present time.

LOCOMOTION

In animals, locomotion is achieved either by movement of the limbs with each limb showing an alternating activity in the flexor and extensor musculature, or by twisting movements of the body, for example, in the movements of snakes or swimming of fish. When an animal uses all four limbs for locomotion, this is known as quadrupedal locomotion, but some primates, including man, assume an upright position of the body and use only two limbs for progression. This bipedal locomotion releases the forelimbs for manipulation for which they are highly developed. Originally the neuronal systems controlling posture and locomotion were considered to be separate and to work separately. Now it is thought that one or more systems interrelate in the control of locomotion. This includes the systems controlling the body's posture and equilibrium and the mechanisms producing the stepping patterns in the limbs.

In quadrupedal locomotion more than one pattern of interlimb stepping can be seen and in the cat several have been described (Miller et al, 1975a). They can be divided into two basic groups; alternate, when homologous limbs move alternately, for example, the pace or trot; and in phase, when homologous limbs move together, for example, the gallop. In the bipedal gait of man, however, only the alternate type of stepping pattern is seen.

In recent years several E.M.G. studies have been made of the muscle activity in the trunk and lower limbs of man during locomotion (Basmajian, 1979; Carlsöö, 1972; Liberson, 1965). They have shown that the alternating activity of flexors and extensors in one limb is seen in the flexors and extensors of the hip and ankle joints only. Because of the bipedal nature of man's locomotion and the need to keep the body upright, it is necessary for the leg to be kept fairly rigid during the support phase. Therefore, the flexor and extensor muscles of the knee joint act together in a stabilising function during stance, and this ability to break up or fractionate mass patterns of flexion and extension in a limb is one of the distinguishing features of the motor control in primates. In the hemiplegic stroke patient, this ability to break up patterns may be lost and the affected leg may only move in total patterns of flexion or extension. These abnormal, or mass movement, patterns are a feature of spasticity.

NEURAL CONTROL OF LOCOMOTION

Studies in cats

Neurophysiological studies on spinal and decerebrate cats (Sherrington, 1910; Brown, 1911) have shown that stepping patterns are generated by the spinal cord. Isolation of the spinal cord by de-afferentation showed that the stepping patterns will also continue without peripheral input. Miller and Van der Meché (1976) have since demonstrated that the isolated spinal cord of the cat is capable of producing all the stepping patterns that have been identified in the intact cat and various models have been suggested for the spinal locomotor generator. Brown (1914) had previously suggested two mutually inhibitory half-centres, one driving the flexors and the other the extensors. The oscillation between flexion and extension was achieved by an undefined property of fatigue in the inhibitory connections. Other suggested models consisted of a closed-loop circuit of interneurones and a pacemaker idea (see Grillner, 1975). Miller and Scott (1977) recently proposed a half-centre model, based on Brown's idea of 1914 but without using the fatigue component to explain the oscillation.

However, although stepping has been shown to be a spinal mechanism, it has been observed that some form of stimulation, either by peripheral input, for example, change of hip angle, or by stimulation of the descending tracts in the midbrain, is necessary to initiate the movements. Studies have shown that the peripheral input can initiate or modify stepping (see Grillner, 1981 for review). This peripheral input may be from joint, muscle or cutaneous receptors, but appears to come mainly from the hip region. Grillner (1975) found that stepping in chronic spinal and decerebrate cats could be initiated by a change of hip angle and also may be affected by loading on the limb. Also the fact that a spinal cat walking on a treadmill can adapt to the speed of the treadmill (Grillner, 1973) suggests that peripheral input may have a modifying effect on the stepping patterns.

Pearson and Duysens (1976) compared the function of segmental reflexes in the control of stepping in cockroaches and cats. In both animals it was found that if leg extension was blocked mechanically during the stance phase, the rhythmic movements of the leg were inhibited, while the rhythm in the other legs was unchanged. Allowing the blocked leg to slowly extend led to initiation of the swing phase. Unloading the limb was also found, in both animals, to be one means of signalling the end of the stance phase. Figure 4.1 shows the effect of prolonged loading of the triceps surae muscle of the ipsilateral hind limb of the cat on the rhythmic activity occurring in the muscle. Activity in the flexor of the same hind limb can be seen to be interrupted, while activity in the extensor is prolonged.

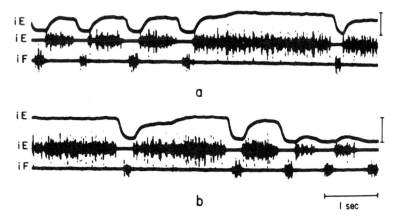

Fig. 4.1 *The effect of prolonged loading of the ipsilateral ankle extensor in a mesencephalic cat walking on a treadmill*

Top traces—force in ankle extensors (calibration = 2.6 kg).

Middle traces—EMG recorded from ipsilateral ankle extensor muscle (triceps surae).

Bottom traces—EMG recorded from ipsilateral ankle flexor muscle (tibialis anterior). (b) is continuous with (a)

Note that during prolonged loading of the ankle extensor there is an abolition of the inhibitory pause in extensor activity and an associated abolition of the flexor burst. Near the end of b the extensor muscle length is reduced and there is a corresponding marked decrease in extensor EMG. (Reprinted from Pearson and Duysens, 1976, with permission from the authors and from Plenum Publishing Corporation, New York.)

While Grillner and Rossignol (1978a) were able to show in experiments with chronic spinal cats that the swing phase could be initiated by extension of the hip joint, the ankle and knee joints did not have the same effect. Anderson et al (1978) also distinguished between hip movements and movements of the knee and ankle joints. They showed that the spinal generator could be 'driven' by hip movement. A new frequency could be imposed on the phasic flexor activity by repeated movements into flexion. Single efferents, identified as belonging to flexors and extensors of the knee and ankle joints, were also recorded in ventral root filaments after the muscles and joints had been denervated. The rhythmic activity in these filaments could also be altered by hip movement. As there was no afferent input from the lower leg, movement of the knee or ankle joint could not be causing the effect.

Cutaneous reflexes have also been shown to have a modifying effect on the spinally generated locomotory patterns. Cutaneous reflexes from the dorsum of the paw of chronic spinal cats walking on a treadmill appear to enhance the activity of the existing state; that is, if a tactile stimulus is applied during stance it enhances the extensor activity, if applied during the swing phase, it enhances the flexor activity (Forssberg et al, 1975; Forssberg et al, 1976). Electrical stimulation of pad and plantar surfaces of the foot in thalamic cats seems to have a similar effect (Duysens & Pearson, 1976). Grillner and Rossignol (1978b) also found that this 'phase dependant reflex reversal' applies to the response to a contralateral stimulus. Duysens (1977) reported slightly different effects from the above by stimulating large (low threshold) and small (high threshold) cutaneous afferents. He suggested that large and small cutaneous afferents make respectively inhibitory and excitatory connections with the spinal generator involved in the generation of flexion during walking. Duysens and Stein (1978) were able to extend this work on the effects of cutaneous reflexes to. normal intact cats with freely moving hind limbs. The results were essentially the same as those reported by Duysens in 1977.

Descending pathways from motor centres in the brain constitute the higher levels of control of locomotion, and many have been found to be phasically active during locomotion in the cat; for example, the lateral vestibulo-spinal tracts show activity in phase with extension, while the rubro-spinal tracts and parts of the reticulo-spinal tracts are active during flexion (Orlovsky, 1970; 1972a and b). It has been shown (Orlovsky, 1972c) that in the decerebrate cat stimulation of the bulbar reticular formation decreases extensor activity during the stance phase but increases the flexor activity during swing. Stimulation of the red nucleus or the pyramidal tracts also increases flexor activity during the swing phase, and stimulation of Deiter's nucleus increases extensor activity during the stance phase. It is not suggested that this phasic activity is necessary to drive the spinal locomotor generator but that the activity may add to the excitation or inhibition of motoneurones and to the force of muscle contraction. However a tonic input does appear to be necessary to start the spinal locomotor generator and the stimulation of a region behind the inferior colliculus, known as the 'mesencephalic locomotor region' (MLR), induces locomotion in the decerebrate cat. It is suggested by Grillner and Shik (1973) that the effects are induced by a slow fibre system that releases the activity of the spinal locomotor generator. Initiation of locomotion by stimulation of the MLR may be due to the stimulation of a locomotor nucleus or to the stimulation of fibre tracts passing through the midbrain. The site of the MLR seems to coincide with the cuneiform nucleus or the brachium conjunctivum (see Mori et al, 1977; Grillner, 1981) but there is also the possibility of other bypassing tracts or nuclei being involved, for example, the nor-adrenergic cell bodies which lie in the locus coeruleus at the rostral end of the fourth ventricle. Stepping can be induced in acute spinal cats by injection of L-dopa or clonidine (Forssberg & Grillner, 1973; Miller & Van der Meché, 1976). These drugs exert their effects on terminals of descending axons from the brainstem that release nor-adrenaline, for example, the reticulospinal pathways from the region of the locus coeruleus and the lower brainstem. Because these pathways are slow fibre systems, Grillner (1976) suggests that it is unlikely that they act as specific initiators of locomotion but they may act to raise the general level of excitability to permit locomotion to take place.

Studies in monkeys

Anatomical and behavioural studies in monkeys (Lawrence & Kuypers, 1968a and b; Kuypers, 1973) also lead to the suggestion that descending motor pathways from the brain may be important for the initiation and modification of basic movement patterns, including stepping, which are generated by the spinal cord. Kuypers (1973), on the basis of the behavioural and anatomical studies, suggests that the descending systems of motor control should be divided into a medial and a lateral division. The medial division appears to be essentially concerned with the control of eye, head, trunk and proximal limb movements. It includes the tecto-spinal and interstitiospinal tracts (from the midbrain), the reticulo-spinal tracts (from the regions of the reticular formation), the vestibulospinal tracts and the ventral corticospinal tracts. This division also seems to be involved in the switching on and off of spinal programmes of movement (Grillner, 1975; Miller et al, 1975b). The lateral division would appear to be concerned mainly with movements of distal parts of the limbs, with fractionation of movement patterns and with fine discrete movements, particularly of the digits. This division includes the corticobulbar tracts (to brainstem nuclei of cranial motor nerves), the lateral corticospinal tracts and the rubrospinal tracts.

The two divisions of the descending motor pathways are so-called because of their relative positions within the brainstem and spinal cord. The majority of the fibres, except the direct cortico-moto-neuronal fibres, terminate in the intermediate zone of the spinal cord on interneurones that lie either medially or laterally. Although details appear to be unclear, it does seem that the cells in the medial part of the intermediate zone send their fibres into the ventro-medial part of the ventral horn, and cells in the lateral part of the intermediate zone send their fibres into the dorso-lateral part of the ventral horn (Kuypers, 1973). The ventro-medial and dorso-lateral areas of the ventral horn contain alpha motoneurones that supply proximal limb and axial muscles and distal limb muscles, respectively. Therefore, it would seem that the medial pathways influence trunk and girdle muscles and the lateral pathways influence intrinsic muscles of the limbs. If conditions in the cat are the same as those in the monkey, then as part of the medial division, the noradrenergic reticulospinal fibres exert their effects mainly on interneurones and alpha motoneurones which supply muscles of the trunk and proximal limb joints. This may explain why peripheral influence on the initiation and modification of the stepping patterns also seems to be directed towards the proximal regions.

Studies in man

It has been observed clinically that the trunk and hip are important in locomotion in man (Bobath, 1980) and following stroke the correct alignment of these areas and correct weight transference appears to affect gait performance in the whole leg. The Bobath approach to rehabilitation of the hemiplegic stroke patient is concerned with inhibition of abnormal mass movement patterns and facilitation of normal fractionated movement patterns. It has been observed by Bobath (1980) that there are 'key-points of control' by which muscle tone and performance in the whole of the limb can be controlled or altered. These 'key-points' are mainly proximal, that is, the hip joint, the shoulder joint, the pelvis and the scapula. In the stroke patient, if the spastic pattern is reversed at the hip and pelvic region by extension of the hip and protraction of the pelvis, the tone in the spastic limb is reduced as evident on passive movement. The patient may then be able to perform a fractionated movement, for example, flexion of the knee while the hip is extended. These fractionated movement patterns, performed while muscle tone is being controlled through the 'key-points' are known as reflex-inhibiting patterns.

Herman et al (1973) and Cook and Cozzens (1976) also emphasise the importance of loading and unloading of the limb and the correct alignment of the trunk for the initiation of gait. Miller and Musa

(1982) measured movements of the hip joint and loading of the limb in normal subjects and in stroke patients during gait. The results showed movements of the hip joint in the sagittal plane in the affected leg of the stroke patients to be significantly lower than those of normal subjects and also that in patients who used a walking aid, loading of the affected leg was also significantly lower. In the study, values for hip joint excursion in the affected leg of the stroke patients were also compared with values obtained from clinical assessments carried out on each of the patients. There was a clear correlation between the assessment values and the total hip excursion, thus suggesting that a reduction in hip movement is associated with a reduction in the patient's functional and motor performance. These observations and studies in man therefore support the results of the animal experiments in indicating the importance of hip movements and limb loading in gait.

Receptors responsible for peripheral control

The animal experiments give little information as to which receptors are responsible for the peripheral control and the receptors may be associated with joint, skin or muscle (Anderson et al, 1978; Rossignol & Gauthier, 1977, 1980). A movement of the hip joint could excite primary and secondary muscle spindle afferents by stretch of the muscle (Roberts, 1978) and could also excite receptors in the joint itself. Carli et al (1979) have recently shown that the cat hip joints contain slowly adapting receptors that respond at all ranges. It is also possible that both these types of receptors, that is, joint and muscle, could be stimulated by loading of the limb.

It has been shown (Hultborn, 1972, 1976) that there is a wide convergence from different primary afferents as well as from descending pathways onto interneurones in spinal reflex pathways to alpha-motoneurones. Lundberg (1979) suggests that the different afferents converging at an interneuronal level, form multisensory reflex feedback systems. He suggests that many of these systems may exist in which afferents of different receptor origin act together in a variety of combinations. In particular, two different classes of reflexes seem to exist from the flexor reflex afferents (FRA). Short-latency reflexes that cause ipsilateral limb flexion and contralateral limb extension are found in the acute spinal cat, but after injection of dopa intravenously late, long-lasting reflexes appear (Andén et al, 1966). It is suggested (see Lundberg, 1979) that the short-latency reflex causes an inhibition of the long latency reflex. Dopa causes a transmitter release from descending nor-adrenergic pathways which inhibit the short-latency reflex pathway.

The long-latency pathway is then released from its inhibitory control. Combined stimulation of ipsilateral and contralateral FRA in the acute spinal cat injected with dopa intravenously reveals a reciprocal organisation in that either flexor or extensor motoneurones are activated (Jankowska et al, 1967). It is, therefore, suggested that the long-latency FRA pathway may play a role in stepping (Lundberg, 1979). It was once considered that the FRA are activated only by strong mechanical nociceptive-like stimuli but Lundberg (1979) suggests that there is some evidence that afferents belonging to this system are activated in normal movements and by passive limb movements in acute spinal cats. If so, then hip movements and limb loading may excite FRA receptors and give a positive feedback during locomotion.

SPASTICITY AND THE TONIC STRETCH REFLEX

The stroke patient with a spastic hemiplegia has lost the ability to break up or fractionate total movement patterns and shows an increase in tone in certain muscle groups. Emphasis on the correct alignment of the hip region and on correct weight transference appears to reduce tone and to inhibit abnormal movement patterns in the lower limb.

Current theories on the physiological mechanisms underlying spasticity suggest that the tonic stretch reflex may play an important part. The tonic stretch reflex is a polysynaptic spinal reflex and in a normal, relaxed subject it is not evident on passive movement or stretch of a muscle. However, a voluntary contraction of the muscle against a passive stretching force elicits the reflex, with the resultant tonic contraction (Lance & McLeod, 1981). In spasticity there is a hyper-activity of the dynamic component of the tonic stretch reflex so that it can be elicited by passive stretch alone. The size of the response to the passive stretching is determined by the velocity of the movement and is therefore said to be velocity sensitive. Neilson (1972) studied the tonic stretch reflex in normal subjects and in patients with spasticity due to cerebral palsy. He found that in the spastic subjects the reflex was in a fully 'switched-on' or hyperactive state at all times. This hyperactivity was presumed to be due to an increase in fusimotor activity or to a disinhibition of spinal pathways associated with the reflex.

Other studies on patients with spasticity (Hagbarth et al, 1973; Hagbarth et al, 1975) have been unable to show any evidence of increased fusimotor activity. Burke (1980), in a review of the current findings concerning the muscle spindle contribution to muscle tone, concludes that evidence so far obtained suggests that the increase in stretch reflex gain seen in patients with spasticity occurs through a central mechanism independent of the fusimotor system.

The tonic vibration reflex (TVR)

Recently, the tonic vibration reflex (TVR) has been used to study tonic spinal reflex mechanisms in both cat and man. Early observations of the TVR (Eklund & Hagbarth, 1966; Mathews, 1966; Brown et al, 1967) showed it to be a tonic reflex contraction of a muscle caused by vibration of muscle spindles inducing activity preferentially and selectively in Ia afferents.

Because this effect can be produced without fusimotor activity, the TVR is a useful tool for studying tonic spinal mechanisms in cat and man and their alteration in spastic man. A supra spinal element seems to be necessary for the TVR (Gillies et al, 1971) and in spinal man it is absent (Hagbarth, 1973; Dimitrijevic et al, 1977). Studies in the cat have shown that it is facilitated from the lateral vestibular nucleus and pontine reticular formation, and inhibited by the medial medullary reticular formation (Gillies et al, 1971). The medullary inhibitory region is facilitated by concomitant stimulation of the motor cortex (Andrews et al, 1973), indicating that it is driven or controlled by the motor cortex. If the situation is the same in man, then a lesion to the corticoreticular connections as they pass through the internal capsule could result in a lack of inhibition of tonic spinal mechanisms, as seen following stroke. When the TVR has been found to occur in the spastic patient it has tended to develop abruptly, unlike the TVR of the normal subject which develops more slowly (Hagbarth & Eklund, 1968; Burke et al, 1972). Normal subjects can voluntarily suppress the TVR, but when this happens there is no sign of a decrease in muscle spindle discharge (Burke et al, 1976). This suggests that this voluntary change in reflex gain is not brought about by an inhibition of fusimotor drive, and therefore it is presumed to be due to an inhibition of central mechanisms. Patients with spasticity are unable to suppress the tonic vibration reflex (Hagbarth & Ekland, 1968; Burke et al, 1972), and therefore it appears that spasticity is associated with the loss of the ability to inhibit central spinal mechanisms associated with the TVR. In the cat and in man, the TVR has been shown to abolish the phasic mono-synaptic reflex while it is activated, and it appears to do this by a process of presynaptic inhibition (Gillies et al, 1968; Dindar & Verrier, 1975; Ashby & Verrier, 1980). In spastic hemiplegia in man, this suppression of the mono-synaptic reflex is reduced and in spinal man it does not take place at all. This led Burke and Ashby (1972) to suggest that presynaptic inhibitory mechanisms may be reduced or lost in spasticity. They postulate that presynaptic inhibitory mechanisms are not irrevocably turned off but deprived of supraspinal support; they are suppressed.

DISCUSSION

The animal experiments described above show that hip movements and limb loading are important for both the initiation and modification of gait and may be responsible for the switching on of the spinal locomotor generator. It is also suggested that hip movements and limb loading may excite FRA receptors and give a positive feedback during locomotion. Lundberg (1979) suggested that the positive feedback from the FRA may be controlled by the descending inhibition of interneurones from the brainstem, but that segmental presynaptic inhibition may also play a role. In support of this he cited the work of Eccles et al (1962) who demonstrated that the FRA evoke primary afferent depolarisation in their own terminals, which suggests a negative feedback control of transmission. It was also suggested by Grillner and Rossignol (1978b) that peripheral activity may have an inhibitory effect on activity in FRA pathways. They suggest that 'the central network for locomotion is effectively driven by a rather unspecific input, and that this input is gated to the 'extensor' and then the 'flexor' parts of the central network, depending at least partially on the position of the limb'.

The studies in man have also led to the conclusion that hip movements and limb loading are important in gait and it is also possible that the spasticity seen in the stroke patient is due to a loss of descending inhibition on spinal reflex pathways and particularly to a loss of presynaptic inhibition. Therefore, if the situation in man is the same as that in the cat then the inability of the stroke patient to perform normal movement patterns, including normal gait patterns, may be due to a lack of inhibition on short-latency FRA pathways. This inhibition may normally be exerted by the noradrenergic reticulospinal pathways but also by segmental presynaptic inhibitory mechanisms. As Burke and Ashby (1972) suggested, the presynaptic inhibitory mechanisms may not be irrevocably switched off but only suppressed due to a loss of their supraspinal support. This supraspinal support may be completely lost, but in the case of an internal capsular lesion there may only be partial damage to cortico-reticular fibres, depending on the extent of the lesion.

The question that needs to be considered is whether the manipulation of peripheral input alone (with little or no supraspinal support) can be sufficient to switch on the presynaptic inhibitory mechanisms so that they are able to exert their effect on the short-latency FRA pathways. Empirical evidence (personal observations; also see Bobath, 1980) so far suggests that alteration of peripheral input, particularly with regard to movements of the hip joint and limb loading, can reduce muscle tone in a spastic limb so that normal gait patterns can be performed. It is possible that this reduction in muscle tone in man may be due to a segmental presynaptic inhibitory mechanism acting on spinal reflex pathways.

FURTHER STUDIES

It is suggested that there is sufficient evidence to justify the use of techniques that concentrate on limb loading and the correct alignment of the hip in the retraining of gait in the spastic hemiplegic stroke patient. However, evidence other than empirical observation is needed to show that muscle tone can be reduced in a limb by manipulation of peripheral input. It may be possible to show by measurement of the H-reflex or the TVR in the spastic hemiplegic stroke patient whether changes in peripheral input cause any alterations in the excitability of central reflex pathways. The H-reflex has so far been used to measure the excitability of monosynaptic pathways and also of different inhibitory mechanisms operating at segmental level in the spinal cord. Yanagisawa et al (1976) used the H-reflex to demonstrate an excessive reciprocal inhibition in the anterior tibial muscles in man when a stimulus was applied to the spastic calf muscles. This excessive inhibition was attributed to a Ia inhibitory mechanism. El-Tohamy and Sedgwick (1983) have investigated a second phase of inhibition which is seen in antagonistic muscles on stimulation of the agonists in normal man. They attribute this second phase of inhibition to activity in Gr. II afferents and they found it to be absent in the spastic soleus muscle of 5 hemiplegic patients (El-Tohamy & Sedgwick, 1982). It may be possible to use the H-reflex to measure any changes occurring in the excitability of central reflex pathways during physiotherapeutic manipulation of peripheral input, and also to measure any long-term changes that may take place.

In the neural control of locomotion, evidence is needed to show more clearly the organisation of the spinal locomotor generator and to show whether such a model exists in man. The generator model suggested by Miller and Scott (1977, 1980) is considered to control a pair of antagonistic muscle groups about a uniaxial joint, for example, the flexors and extensors at the knee joint. Co-ordination of flexor and extensor movements throughout the whole limb is then achieved by the coupling of several generators. Observations of the patterns of muscle activity in the limbs of the cat during locomotion suggest a close coupling of generators, i.e. the onset of extension at one joint being very close in time to the onset of extension in another joint. It is possible that man may possess a greater ability to alter the coupling of generators, i.e. to dissociate flexion and extension movements at different joints. This situation is suggested by the observations made by Miller et al (1978) in comparing forward and backward stepping in man. In spastic man, the ability to dissociate the movements at the different joints and therefore to produce a fractionated movement pattern is lost. Therefore in man, although the situation may be basically the same as that in the cat, i.e. a central pattern generator which can be switched on by descending influence from the brain or by peripheral input, it would also have to be much more complex to allow for man's ability to produce fractionated patterns of movement during locomotion and to show variability in a greater number of parameters during walking and running (see Grillner et al, 1979).

EVALUATION AND RETRAINING OF GAIT FOLLOWING STROKE

As shown by Miller and Musa (1982) movements of the hip joint are reduced in the sagittal plane in the affected leg of stroke patients and this is associated with a reduction in the patient's overall motor and functional ability. In view of it's proven significance, this parameter should provide a useful means of evaluating gait and also the patient's overall functional ability. Limb loading was also found by Miller and Musa (1982) to be reduced in the affected leg of stroke patients who walked with either a walking stick or a tripod or quadrupod type of walking aid. As limb loading has also been shown in animals and man to be significant in the initiation and modification of gait, it should also be an important consideration in gait retraining and in the evaluation of gait. As well as measures of peak loading and total hip movement, patterns of change of these features should also be useful in gait evaluation. Dewar and Judge (1980) distinguished between 'diagnostic' and 'monitoring' types of gait analysis. In the 'monitoring' type, emphasis is placed on a simple, representative measure of gait, while in the 'diagnostic' type emphasis is placed on the measurement of a feature that is important in the diagnosis of a patient's particular condition. Following stroke, a monitoring type of gait analysis, such as a measure of temporal assymetry, would give an overall measure of the patient's gait. Measurements of limb loading and hip movements as well as giving this overall measure of gait would also provide a quantitative and a qualitative measure of the patient's progress with regard to the natural history of stroke. They would also give useful indications for treatment.

Miller and Musa (1982) suggested a method of combining the cyclical changes of hip excursion and limb loading during gait, by combining them for display in X–Y plots. Characteristic patterns for the limbs of normal subjects and stroke patients have been obtained (see Fig. 4.2), and they would provide a meaningful reference for evaluation.

In the retraining of gait following stroke, treatment approaches that attempt to establish normal ranges of hip joint movement and loading of the limb should be the most efficacious. In particular, patients who use a walking stick or another form of walking aid will not load the affected leg fully. Figure 4.2d shows the X–Y plot from the affected leg of a right-sided hemiplegic patient who walked with an aid. The limb is only being loaded to approximately 80% of body weight during the stance phase. Figure 4.3a shows a left-sided hemiplegic stroke patient standing with the aid of a tripod walking aid. The level of the patient's shoulders and the creases on her dress show that most of the body weight is being exerted either through the unaffected leg or through the walking aid. However, if the walking aid is removed (Fig. 4.3b), the patient is able to achieve a more symmetrical posture with more equal distribution of weight between the limbs. Re-education of limb loading and weight transference between the limbs can be achieved in the stroke patient by conventional methods but also can be assisted by the use of electronic biofeedback aids. A simple limb load shoe has been used by the author and has been found to be useful.

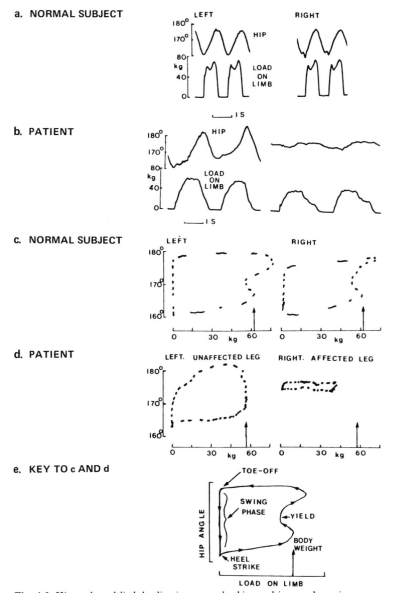

Fig. 4.2 *Hip angle and limb loading in a normal subject and in a stroke patient*
(Right hemiplegia; 3 months post stroke)
   (a) and (b)—raw data
   (c) and (d)—XY plots of hip angle against limb loading; only the first step
shown in the raw data (a and b) has been displayed. Gaps in the trace indicate
time marks at 20 Hz.
   (e)—Key to plots (c) and (d) (Miller & Musa, 1982).

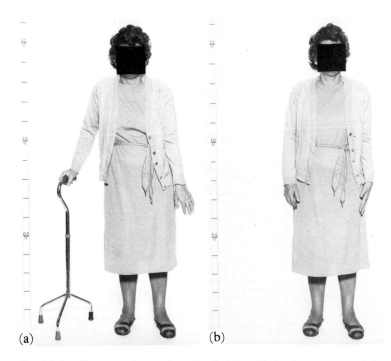

(a)   (b)

Fig. 4.3 *Standing posture in a stroke patient* (Left hemiplegia; 2 years post stroke)
(a)—Standing with the aid of a tripod walking aid: most of the body weight is being exerted either through the unaffected leg or through the walking aid.
(b)—When the walking aid is removed the patient is able to stand unaided and exerts more weight through the affected leg.

In summary, this chapter has reviewed the recently published literature on the neural control of locomotion and on the neurophysiology of spasticity, and has sought to relate the current ideas to the clinical situation seen in the spastic hemiplegic stroke patient. It is suggested that while further studies are needed to clarify the situation, methods of gait re-education that seek to achieve correct alignment of the hip joint and loading of the affected limb should be preferred and should prove efficacious. Also these parameters should provide useful criteria for the evaluation of recovery of normal gait following stroke.

REFERENCES

Andén N E, Jukes M G M, Lundberg A, Vyklicky L 1966 The effect of dopa on the spinal cord. I. Influence on transmission from primary afferents. Acta Physiologica Scandinavica 67: 373–386

Anderson O, Grillner S, Lindquist M, Zomlefer M 1978 Peripheral control of the spinal pattern generators for locomotion in cat. Brain Research 150: 625–630

Andrews C, Knowles L, Lance J W 1873 Corticoreticulospinal control of the tonic vibration reflex in the cat. Journal of the Neurological Sciences 18: 207–216

Ashby P, Verrier M 1980 Human motoneurone responses to group I volleys blocked presynaptically by vibration. Brain Research 184: 511–516

Basmajian J V 1979 Muscles alive. Williams and Wilkins, Baltimore

Bobath B 1980 Adult hemiplegia: evaluation and treatment. Heinemann, London

Brown T G 1911 The intrinsic factor in the act of progression in the mammal. Proceedings of the Royal Society B84: 308–319

Brown T G 1914 On the nature of the fundamental activity of the nervous centres; together with an analysis of the conditioning of rhythmic activity in progression, and a theory of the evolution of function in the nervous system. Journal of Physiology 48: 18–46

Brown M C, Engberg I, Mathews P B C 1967 The relative sensitivity to vibration of muscle receptors of the cat. Journal of physiology 192: 773–800

Brunnström S 1970 Movement therapy in hemiplegia. Harper and Row, New York

Burke D 1980 A reassessment of the muscle spindle contribution to muscle tone in normal and spastic man. In: Feldman R G, Young R R, Koella W P (eds) Spasticity: disordered motor control. Year Book Medical Publications, Chicago, p 261–278

Burke D, Ashby P 1972 Are spinal 'presynaptic' inhibitory mechanisms suppressed in spasticity. Journal of the Neurological Sciences 15: 321–326

Burke D, Andrews C J, Lance J W 1972 Tonic vibration reflex in spasticity, Parkinson's disease and normal subjects. Journal of neurology, neurosurgery and psychiatry 35: 447–486

Burke D, Hagbarth K E, Lofstedt L, Wallin B G 1976 The responses of human muscle spindle endings to vibration during isometric contraction. Journal of Physiology 261: 695–711

Carli G, Farabollini F, Fontani G, Meucci M 1979 Slowly adapting receptors in cat hip joint. Journal of Neurophysiology 42: 767–778

Carlsoo S 1972 How man moves. Heinemann, London

Cook T, Cozzens B 1976 Human solutions for locomotion: III The initiation of gait. In: Herman R M, Grillner S, Stein P S G, Stuart D G (eds) Neural control of locomotion. Plenum Publishing Corporation, New York, p 65–77

Dewar M E, Judge G 1980 Temporal asymmetry as a gait quality indicator. Medical and Biological Engineering and Computing 18: 689–693

Dimitrijevic M R, Spencer W A Trontelj J V, Dimitrejevic M 1977 Reflex effects of vibration in patients with spinal cord lesions. Neurology 27: 1078–1086

Dindar F, Verrier M 1975 Studies on the receptor responsible for vibration induced inhibition of monosynaptic reflexes in man. Journal of neurology, neurosurgery and psychiatry 38: 155–160

Duysens J 1977 Reflex control of locomotion as revealed by stimulation of cutaneous afferents in spontaneously walking premammillary cats. Journal of Neurophysiology 40: 737–751

Duysens J, Pearson K G 1976 The role of cutaneous afferents from the distal hindlimb in the regulation of the step cycle of thalamic cats. Experimental Brain Research 24: 245–255

Duysens J, Stein R B 1978 Reflexes induced by nerve stimulation in walking cats with implanted cuff electrodes. Experimental Brain Research 32: 213–224

Eccles J C, Kostyuk P G, Schmidt R F 1962 Presynaptic inhibition of the central actions of flexor reflex afferents. Journal of Physiology 161: 258–281

Eklund G, Hagbarth K E 1966 Normal variability of tonic vibration reflexes in man. Experimental Neurology 16: 80–92

El-Tohamy A, Sedgwick E M 1982 Spinal inhibitory mechanisms in spasticity. Electroencephalography and Clinical Neurophysiology 53: 1–49

El-Tohamy A, Sedgwick E M 1983 Spinal inhibition in man: depression of the soleus H reflex by stimulation of the nerves to the antagonist muscle. Journal of Physiology 337: 497–508

Forssberg H, Grillner S 1973 The locomotion of the acute spinal cat injected with clonidine i.v. Brain Research 50: 184–186

Forssberg H, Grillner S, Rossignol S 1975 Phase dependent reflex reversal during walking in chronic spinal cats. Brain Research 85: 103–107

Forssberg H, Grillner S, Rossignol S, Wallén P 1976 Phasic control of reflexes during locomotion in vertebrates. In: Herman R M, Grillner S, Stein P S G, Stuart D G (eds) Neural control of locomotion. Plenum Publishing Corporation, New York, p 647–674

Gillies J D, Burke D J, Lance J W 1971 Supraspinal control of tonic vibration reflex. Journal of Neurophysiology 34: 302–309

Gillies J D, Lance J W, Neilson P D, Tassinari C A 1969 Presynaptic inhibition of the monosynaptic reflex. Journal of Physiology 205: 329–339

Grillner S 1973 On the spinal generation of locomotion. In: Batuer A S (ed) Sensory organisation of movements. Leningrad

Grillner S 1975 Locomotion in vertebrates: Central mechanisms and reflex interaction. Physiological Reviews 55: 247–304

Grillner S 1976 Some aspects on the descending control of the spinal circuits generating locomotor movements. In: Herman R M, Grillner S, Stein P S G, Stuart D G (eds) Neural control of locomotion. Plenum Publishing Corporation, New York, p 351–375

Grillner S 1981 Control of locomotion in bipedes, tetra-podes and fish. In: Brooks V (ed) Handbook of physiology Volume III, Section I. The nervous system II Motor control. American Physiological Society, Waverley Press, Baltimore, p 1179–1236

Grillner S, Rossignol S 1978a On the initiation of the swing phase of locomotion in chronic spinal cats. Brain Research 146: 269–277

Grillner S, Rossignol S 1978b Contralateral reflex reversal controlled by limb position in the acute spinal cat injected with clonidine i.v. Brain Research 144: 411–414

Grillner S, Shik M L 1973 On the descending control of the lumbosacral spinal cord from the 'mesencephalic locomotor region'. Acta Physiologica Scandinavica 87: 320–333

Grillner S, Halbertsma J, Nilsson J, Thorstensson A 1979 The adaptation to speed in human locomotion. Brain Research 165: 177–182

Hagbarth K-E 1973 The effect of muscle vibration in normal man and in patients with motor disorders. In: Desmedt J E (ed) New developments in EMG and clinical neurophysiology, Volume 3. Karger, Basel, p 428–443

Hagbarth K-E, Eklund G 1968 The effects of muscle vibration in spasticity, rigidity and cerebellar disorders. Journal of Neurology, Neurosurgery and Psychiatry 31: 207–213

Hagbarth K-E, Wallin G, Lofstëdt L 1973 Muscle spindle responses to stretch in normal and spastic subjects. Scandinavian Journal of Rehabilitation Medicine 5: 156–159

Hagbarth K-E, Wallin G, Lofstëdt L, Aquilonius S-M 1975 Muscle spindle activity in alternating tremor of Parkinsonism and in clonus. Journal of Neurology, Neurosurgery and Psychiatry 38: 625–635 and 636–641

Herman R, Cook T, Cozzens B, Freedman W 1973 Control of postural reactions in man: The initiation of gait. In: Stein R B, Pearson K G, Smith R S, Redford J B (eds) Control of posture and locomotion. Plenum Publishing Corporation, New York, p 363–388

Hultborn H 1972 Convergence on interneurones in the reciprocal Ia inhibitory pathway to motoneurones. Acta Physiologica Scandinavica 85: supplement 375 p 1–42

Hultborn H 1976 Transmission in the pathway of reciprocal Ia inhibition to motoneurones and it's control during the tonic stretch reflex. Progress in Brain Research 44: 235–256

Jankowska E, Jukes M G M, Lund S, Lundberg A 1967 The effect of dopa on the spinal cord. 5. Reciprocal organisation of pathways transmitting excitatory action to alpha motoneurones of flexors and extensors. Acta Physiologica Scandinavica 70: 369–388

Kuypers H G J M 1973 The anatomical organisation of the descending pathways and their contribution to motor control especially in primates. In: Desmedt J E (ed) New developments in EMG and clinical neurophysiology, Volume 3, Karger, Basal p 38–68

Lance J W, McLeod J G 1981 A physiological approach to clinical neurology. Butterworth, London

Lawrence D G, Kuypers H J G M 1968a The functional organisation of the motor system in the monkey. I. The effects of bilateral pyramidal lesions. Brain 91: 1–14

Lawrence D G, Kuypers H J G M 1968b The functional organization of the motor system in the monkey. 2. The effects of lesions of the descending brain-stem pathways. Brain 91: 15–33

Liberson W T 1965 Biomechanics of gait: A method of study. Archives of Physical Medicine 46: 37–48

Lundberg A 1979 Multisensory control of spinal reflex pathways. Progress in Brain Research 50: 11–28

Mathews P B C 1966 The reflex excitation of the soleus muscle of the decerebrate cat caused by vibration applied to its tendon. Journal of Physiology 184: 450–472

Miller S, Musa I M 1982 The significance of hip movement and vertical loading on the foot in the evaluation and retraining of gait in stroke patients. Proceedings of the IXth. WCPT International Congress p 765–771

Miller S, Scott P D 1977 The spinal locomotor generator. Experimental Brain Research 30: 387–403

Miller S, Scott P D 1980 Spinal generation of movement in a single limb: functional implications of a model based on the cat. In: Desmedt J E (ed) Progress in clinical neurophysiology, Volume 8. Karger, Basel, p 263–281

Miller S, van der Meché F G A 1976 Co-ordinated stepping of all four limbs in the high spinal cat. Brain Research 109: 395–398

Miller S, Mitchelson D, Scott P D 1978 Coupling of hip and knee movement during forward and backward stepping in man. Journal of Physiology 277: 45–46P

Miller S, van der Burg J, van der Meché F G A 1975a Co-ordination of movements of the hindlimbs and forelimbs in different forms of locomotion in normal and decerebrate cats. Brain Research 91: 217–237

Miller S, van der Burg J, van der Meché F G A 1975b Locomotion in the cat: basic programmes of movement. Brain Research 91: 239–253

Mori S, Shik M L, Yagodnitsyn A S 1977 Role of pontine tegmentum for locomotor control in mesencephalic cat. Journal of Neurophysiology 40: 284–295

Neilson P D 1972 Interaction between voluntary contraction and tonic stretch reflex transmission in normal and spastic patients. Journal of Neurology, Neurosurgery and Psychiatry. 35: 853–860

Orlovsky G N 1970 Work of the reticulo-spinal neurones during locomotion. Biofizika 15: 728–737

Orlovsky G N 1972a Activity of vestibulospinal neurones during locomotion. Brain Research 46: 85–98

Orlovsky G N 1972b Activity of rubrospinal neurones during locomotion. Brain Research 46: 99–112

Orlovsky G N 1972c The effect of different descending system on flexor and extensor activity during locomotion. Brain Research 40: 359–371

Pearson K G, Duysens J 1976 Function of segmental reflexes in the control of stepping in cockroaches and cats. In: Herman R M, Griller S, Stein P S G, Stuart D G (eds) Neural control of locomotion. Plenum Publishing Corporation, New York, p 519–535

Perry J 1980 Rehabilitation of spasticity. In: Feldman R G, Young R R, Koella W P (eds) Spasticity: disordered motor control. Year book medical publications, Chicago p 87–100

Rossignol S, Gauthier L 1977 Reversal of contralateral limb reflexes. Proceedings of the International Union of the Physiological Sciences 13:639

Rossignol S, Gauthier L 1980 An analysis of mechanisms controlling the reversal of crossed spinal reflexes. Brain Research 182: 31–45

Roberts T D M 1978 Neurophysiology of Postural Mechanisms. Butterworths, London

Sherrington C S 1910 Flexion-reflex of the limb, crossed extension-reflex and reflex stepping and standing. Journal of Physiology 40: 28–121

Yanagisawa N, Tanaka R, Ito Z 1976 Reciprocal Ia inhibition in spastic hemiplegia of man. Brain 99: 555–574

A neuro-physiological approach

INTRODUCTION

Modern concepts of neuro-muscular physiology and of plasticity of the system have much to offer in the rehabilitation of stroke patients. This chapter deals mainly with the development of Miss Margaret Rood's concept of physical treatment. Writing in 1956 Rood recognised that a knowledge of the differences in fast and slow skeleto-motor units was significant and should influence the choice of stimuli applied by therapists to elicit motor activity or to inhibit unwanted phenomenon. Her concept is applicable to many clinical manifestations of the consequences of cerebrovascular disease, including cases with sensory or perceptual defects, apraxia or problems of communication.

It should also be noted that many stimuli and techniques are effective even if the patient is unconscious. In 1956 Rood wrote: 'Muscles have different duties. Most of them are a combination but some predominate in "light-work" others in "heavy-work"'. This difference in the work done by muscles with different enzyme profiles is fully supported by researchers in neuro-physiology. Burke (1980) noted that: 'In summary the evidence suggests that the difference between the motor unit types represent specialisations that are matched quite exactly to the functional demands placed on the muscle in which they are found'. So, it is for the therapist to select appropriate stimuli which will activate muscles to fulfil the functional demands needed to achieve motor goals. For example: stimuli which maintain posture and elicit normal postural reactions, repeated over a sufficient period of time, inform the central nervous system (C.N.S.) of the demands of the musculo-skeletal system. Trophic changes then occur in muscle and nerve and facilitate future motor behaviour.

The term 'plasticity' is used to indicate that nerve and muscle tissue are not permanently fixed in form or function but, by trophic influences, can eventually change at molecular level to meet new demands. This concept offers an exciting challenge to physiotherapists to select, apply and repeat stimuli which will bring about trophic changes. Motor units suited to the activity demanded will hypertrophy. More significantly, where damage or disease necessitates adaptation, changes may be promoted so that motor units shift over to a type better suited to the needs of the patient. That is, muscle and nerve not only become more efficient if used in ways for which they are designed, but can adapt to fulfil a new role if appropriate demands on them are made. Rood's concept recognises that afferent input can profoundly influence the type of muscle work performed.

Motor unit types

Rood refers to muscles as doing 'light-work' or 'heavy-work'. Researchers classify skeleto-motor units as phasic or tonic and several classifications are used in the literature. One classification which is used by Kidd & Brodie (1980) when listing the characteristics of skeletal muscle fibres is based upon metabolic and mechanical properties. Three types are described—Slow Oxidative (S.O.), Fast Glycolytic (F.G), and Fast Oxidative Glycolytic (F.O.G.). A muscle such as soleus consists mainly of S.O. motor units and corresponds to that which Rood recognises as doing 'heavy-work'. In contrast, a muscle such as gastrocnemius, a multiarthrodial muscle, consists mainly of F.G. motor units and does 'light-work'.

Kidd (1980) wrote: 'These classes are not immutable'. Their relative differences can become less distinct when, for example, the intermediate (F.O.G.) fibres change in character away from one extreme towards the other. Or the differences between them become more distinct if the outline of what is described as their individual enzyme profile becomes more pronounced. When S.O. muscle fibres experience increased motor activity of a kind for which their metabolic and mechanical properties are suitable, adaptation leads to an increase in the number, size and complexity of their mitochondria. The consequent increase in capacity for oxidative metabolism induces capillarisation of the muscle fibres, appropriately enhancing their blood supply. When motor units are involved in prolonged activity inappropriate to their class, the muscle fibres also adapt and they do so by changing to a state better suited to the enforced activity.

Unfortunately, pathological states often have a profound and rapid influence on trophic changes within the neuro-muscular system. Thus clinical phenomena, such as spasticity, decerebrate rigidity or other disorders of muscle tone are reinforced. All forms of therapy, medical and paramedical, need to be directed towards preventing unwanted plastic changes, and it appears that it is more likely that F.G. motor units will adapt towards the S.O. class than vice versa (Kidd, 1983).

FUNDAMENTALS

Ontogenetic sequences

An awareness of the normal sequence of development in the maturing neuro-muscular system guides the choice of activity, so ensuring an adequate postural background before fine skilled movements are expected.

Rood considers, first, a total movement pattern of flexion; curling up with flexion of head, trunk and limbs, or total extension or rolling. These are very early movement patterns in a baby and so offer a major facilitation to any component of the pattern. They are facilitated by stimuli, assisted if necessary or omitted if not desirable. The total flexion and extension activities require bilateral symmetrical components and in a case of stroke the unaffected side will facilitate the affected one. However, if extensor spasticity is present total extension is omitted.

When total movements have been elicited, a good postural background of stability of head, trunk, proximal and intermediate limb joints is obtained by fixing the distal segment of the part. Compression is given in the long axis of the segment in correct alignment for weight bearing. The choice of position of the whole body and of the part(s) supporting weight is carefully selected, being convenient, comfortable and of immediate functional use to the patient. The part must be supported until the deep muscles are felt to be working. At the same time compression is given so that the weight taken is greater than the weight of the part. Information is thus given to the CNS, demanding cocontraction of slow-acting motor units in deep postural muscles.

When stability is achieved proximally, movement is given of body weight over the fixed distal part. This prepares for mobile stability needed to control a body segment and allows fine precise selective movements to achieve a motor goal. The supporting surface can be moved under the patient or the patient can move over the support whilst keeping the distal end fixed. An example of such an activity is rocking backwards and forwards or sideways over a fixed forearm in a forearm-supporting position.

Finally, precise movements with the distal end of the part free are elicited by motivation. These include precise arm movements, normal sequence of gait and tongue and lip movement for speech.

Stimuli

Many types of stimuli are used and it is important for therapists to understand that these can produce desired effects even if the patient is unconscious, unwilling or unable to co-operate. Afferent impulses reach the spinal cord, brain-stem, cerebellum and many centres in the cerebrum and produce responses without conscious co-operation from the patient. Writing on the treatment of unconscious patients to improve respiratory function and using Rood's methods Bethune (1975) stated: 'Patients' chests are auscultated before, during and after treatment. Changes, increases, in air entry are noted with all procedures'.

As each type of stimulation is discussed it will be explained which need sensory awareness or some motor control to be effective and which do not. Stimulation which is used to excite receptors sensitive to changes in external and internal environment is given to skin, muscles, tendons, mechano-receptors in joints and fascia, to bone and to the labyrinth. Although methods to do so will be discussed separately for each type of stimulation, in treatment many combinations are used.

Cutaneous stimulation

(i) *Fast brushing*. This is applied lightly, quickly with a soft brush or the fingertips to very specific areas of skin. The root nerve supply is the same as that of the muscle to be facilitated and the skin and muscle must be on the same surface of the part. The afferent input from the receptors in the skin increases fusimotor impulses to the muscle spindles, so increasing their sensitivity. There is a delay in the effect so it is done up to twenty minutes before other stimuli are used, thus gaining maximal benefit. If successful regimes of treatment are repeated frequently, brushing will be effective with a shorter delay than is at first needed, and eventually will not be necessary. Brushing is not continued in one place for more than a few seconds.

An added benefit, in cases of spastic hypertonicity, is that the fusimotor input is reduced to the antagonists of the muscles being facilitated. For example, brushing for the anterior fibres of deltoid will both facilitate those and inhibit the posterior fibres and the retractors of the shoulder girdle. Brushing to skin supplied by anterior primary rami of spinal nerves has major effect on superficial muscles whereas brushing to skin supplied by posterior primary rami has an effect on deep muscles of the vertebral column. For most muscles the overlying skin has the same nerve root supply as its motor nerve(s) but as this is not invariable this must be checked (Goff, 1972). Support for the rationale is inconclusive, but in 1980 Leob & Hoffer wrote: 'New data are presented demonstrating that cutaneous afferent stimulation causes rapid and large modulation of muscle spindle activity presumably through complex gamma motoneuron reflexes'.

(*ii*) *Slow stroking.* This is applied from the neck to sacrum over the centre of the back. As one hand reaches the base of the spine the other commences at the neck. Slow rhythmical strokes are applied for three minutes. The effect is to reduce the central excitatory state of neuronal sets of lower motor neurones in the brain stem and spinal cord. Hyperactive flexor spasms may be reduced in this way. Side lying is a suitable position for the patient. This technique should be used with caution in cases with extensor hypertonicity and avoided if it causes increased tone. It is useful in some cases of dystonia but must not be used for patients in a comotosed state.

(*iii*) *Cold* is also applied to the skin by means of an ice cube. The skin is stroked lightly and quickly, but cold drips must not be allowed to spread to areas not required. It is used specifically over the skin with the same nerve root supply as the muscle to be facilitated, has an immediate facilitatory effect and the major facilitation is to extensors and abductors. Cold application is avoided to any area supplied by posterior primary rami of spinal nerves (Goff, 1969).

Cold applied to the lips or to the palmer surface of the fingertips has a stimulating effect on the brain and increases awareness of the part touched. It may, however, increase spasticity of the hand and therefore should be used with caution on the fingertips.

Its application to the lips is used to improve articulation. It is convenient to use plain water frozen in an ice-lollipop form as it can be sucked by the patient. This also facilitates swallowing.

Skin stimulation by any of the three methods described above is effective even if cutaneous sensation is impaired or absent. If the lesion is other than in the peripheral sensory neurones the nerve impulses generated may not reach the sensorium but they do affect the excitability of the lower motor neuronal sets in the ventral grey column of brain-stem and spinal cord. In patients with left-sided neglect, body image defects or other perceptual defects, light quick brushings over all aspects of the affected limbs improves awareness.

Cold applied to the fingertips has a stimulating effect and also improves awareness. The beneficial effect is enhanced by subsequently applying other stimuli to elicit postural reactions.

Stretch

(i) *Slow stretch* applied slowly and fully and maintained for five minutes or more is used to lengthen deep postural muscles, care being taken not to stretch muscles passing over two or more joints. This procedure adjusts the sensitivity to stretch of the muscle spindles in slow-acting motor units. For example, to lengthen the soleus muscle the calf is slowly stretched with the knee flexed, care being taken not to give sudden pressure on the ball of the foot. The heel is grasped and gently pulled down so dorsi-flexing the ankle. Any convenient starting position can be used; crook lying, side lying or prone lying. It can be achieved by the patient in sitting, following instruction in the correct technique. The explanation offered by physiologists is that secondary endings on intrafusal muscle fibres in muscle spindles of deep uniarthrodial muscles are stimulated; the inflow from these to the C.N.S. has an inhibitory effect on the fusimotor flow to the muscle in which they lie and a facilitatory effect on fusimotor flow to their antagonists. Boyd (1980) wrote 'present work confirms the long accepted view that the secondary ending is a length measuring device which derives most input from nuclear chain fibres'. Hunt et al (1960) found 'that group II afferents (from secondary endings in muscle spindles) produce reflex inhibition in extensors and excitation in flexors'. Applying this rationale to a slow stretch of soleus, this muscle would therefore be inhibited and the dorsiflexors facilitated. The facilitation and activation of the dorsiflexors then produces an inhibitory effect on their antagonistic long muscle, the gastrocnemius. Valbo et al (1979) stated: 'the I a afferents (from muscle spindles) have inhibitory projections to antagonistic motor neurons'. The net result should be that the foot can be brought to a right angle with the knee straight, allowing a correct weight bearing standing position. In most stroke patients the spastic foot is inverted as well as plantar flexed. To overcome this the foot is held in eversion and dorsiflexion as the calf is stretched, thus the medial part of the soleus is inhibited and the toe extensors and evertors are facilitated.

The technique of slow stretch is useful in the reduction of tone in any postural muscle, e.g. posterior deltoid, retractors or shoulder girdle, the vasti, hip abductors or deep neck and back muscles. This technique requires neither any sensory awareness nor volitional control by the patient.

Multiarthrodial muscles do not respond favourably to this technique, possibly because there are few, if any, secondary endings in their muscle spindles. Most large muscles contain some motor units of each type, so evaluation of techniques used is essential to ensure improvement. However some groups of muscles, mainly adductors of hip and gleno-humeral joint, do respond to a technique to lengthen multiarthrodial muscles in spite of some components of the group passing over only one joint. The technique for inhibition of multiarthrodial muscle is described below in the section on non-resisted, repeated, volitional movements in small range.

(ii) *Quick stretch* is facilitatory for all types of motor units so should be avoided in lesions of the cortico-spinal system.

Non-resisted, repeated, volitional movements in small range

This technique aims to stimulate the golgi-tendon organ at musculo-tendonous junctions. There is much discussion in the literature on the role of the golgi-tendon organ; two populations are now recognised—one at the musculo-tendonous junction, the other at the tendo-osseous junction.

Kidd wrote (1980) 'The golgi-tendon organ is not a stretch receptor, it is a force receptor.' More exactly, it is able to discriminate between the force applied to a muscle (i.e. by stretching it) and the force engendered in a muscle by its own contraction. The golgi organs are so distributed along the force vectors of the muscle that the contractions of every motor unit is continually monitored. The activity of the tendon organ is reflected upon the motor neurons via inhibitory intrinsic neurons.

Matthews (1973) writing on the role of the golgi organ with Ib afferent fibre states 'that such a restrictive view (that it only inhibits contraction when tension on it is excessive) was never very convincing and it has now been abandoned following the demonstration that the amount of tension required to excite tendon organs is invariably quite small in relation to the potential strength of a muscle.'

Haase et al (1975) wrote 'surprising too is the genuine post-synaptic inhibition regularly produced by contraction of an unloaded flexor muscle. Of all the receptors which could conceivably inhibit homonymous and synergic alpha motoneurons all, except perhaps the golgi-tendon organs, can be ruled out'. A further reference to the inhibitory effect of input from golgi-tendon organs is made by Tracey (1980). He wrote: 'These synaptic potentials (evoked by the Ib fibres of golgi-tendon organs) act to inhibit motorneurons of the muscles containing the tendon organs, and excite antagonist motorneurons'. To effect this the patient must be able to co-operate and perform small range movements many times in succession without facilitation or assistance. The part is supported so that resistance from gravity does not occur. Any form of facilitation must be avoided as excitatory stimuli would cancel the inhibitory effect. Even counting or reminding the patient to keep moving should not be used. Auto-inhibition from the golgi-receptors should be summated. These receptors are known as contraction receptors because when the muscle contracts they generate a flow of impulses which have an inhibitory effect on the motoneurone pool supplying the contracting muscle. The small movements must be repeated many times and are then followed by suitable techniques and vocal commands to facilitate the antagonists. Range is thus gained in tight or spastic muscles. The technique is effective in the reduction of spasticity in hip adductors, elbow, wrist and finger flexors. It is, however, quite difficult for the patient who must be able to concentrate and continue to the point of boredom.

Flexors, adductors and multiarthrodial muscles are rich in these receptors which are less numerous or absent in unarthrodial muscles such as extensors or abductors. It follows that although the small movements need contraction alternately of flexors and their antagonists, the former will be inhibited but not the latter. Stimuli used to facilitate extension or weight bearing are used after the above technique. These will be discussed below.

Compression and pressure

Proprioceptive input from mechanoreceptors in joints, dermis and fascia elicits cocontraction of deep postural muscles, especially of spine, proximal and intermediate joints. Wyke (1972), writing on the type, distribution and function of receptors in joints, stated: 'Type I receptors appear to be more densely distributed in the proximal (limb) joints, whilst in the spine they appear to be more numerous in relation to the apophyseal joints of the cervical region than elsewhere'. He continued: 'Physiologically the type I receptors behave as low threshold, slowly adapting mechanoreceptors responding to the changing mechanical stresses obtaining in the part of the fibrous capsule in which they lie. For this reason a proportion of the lowest threshold Type I receptors in each joint capsule is always active in every position of the joint, *even when it is immobile*. The type I receptors may thus be categorised as static and dynamic mechanoreceptors whose discharge pattern signals static joint position, *intra-articular* or *atmospheric pressure changes*, and the direction, amplitude and velocity of the joint movements produced actively or passively. Mechanoreceptor reflex effects on muscle tone are exerted by afferent discharges from both Type I and Type II receptors, the former being of greater clinical importance in influencing posture and gait than the latter.'

This author further stated: 'Serious attention must therefore be given by clinicians—and not least by physiotherapists—to the role of articular reflexes in the regulation of normal and abnormal posture'. To inhibit spasticity, pain or protective muscle spasm and to elicit proximal joint stability so normalising postural muscle tone, pressure is applied to the normal weight-bearing surfaces. Ensuring that alignment of the segments, head, neck and trunk, or of a limb, is correct for weight bearing, compression is given through the long axis of the part. Correctly applied and maintained until the proximal muscles are seen or felt to be working to maintain the position and support body weight, the technique inhibits spasticity, pain or protective muscle spasm. Pressure and compression can be applied by the therapist at the distal end of a correctly positioned part or can be given as it takes weight on a supporting surface. Examples of application to reduce spasticity in the upper limb are as follows:

(i) Ensure correct alignment of the head of humerus in the glenoid cavity and rub firmly along the posterior border of the ulna. This area normally takes weight in the forearm support position. Apply compression from below the forearm to the shoulder. Ask the patient to push the forearm away from the body. When the therapist feels contraction in rotator cuff muscles the arm can be placed in forearm support and compression given from shoulder to forearm.

(ii) To facilitate weight bearing on an extended arm the same care is taken to ensure correct alignment at the gleno-humeral joint. Inhibitory techniques are used to reduce spasticity in the arm and are followed by pressure on the heel of the hand, especially on the ulnar side under the pisiform. Compression is given through the extended arm from the heel of the hand to the shoulder, and when cocontraction is obtained the arm can be used to reach, push or for weight bearing with hand support. Any suitable starting position can be used, and sensory or body image defects do not negate the effectiveness of these techniques, which indeed improve awareness of the part.

An example in the lower limb is, following the use of techniques to inhibit spasticity in the calf, the application of pressure under the medial side of the heel. This facilitates control of the knee and ankle for weight bearing on a plantigrade foot. The foot is placed correctly for weight bearing and compression given from knee to foot. Activities such as bridging, rising from sitting to standing and weight transferring from one buttock to the other whilst sitting, are facilitated by pressure down from hip to foot as the activity is practised.

Positioning with extensor aspect uppermost

Holding a part so that the extensors resist the force of gravity facilitates automatic postural stability. Sitting with the head and trunk unsupported leaning forwards with the spine extended is easy to maintain, but a similar position leaning backwards is difficult, fatiguing and demands cortical concentration. The mechanoreceptors in joints play a vital role in postural reactions. Wyke, writing in 1972, stated: 'Afferent discharges from the receptors in joint tissues also exert potent reflex influences on the activity of the limbs, paravertebral and respiratory musculature at spinal and brain stem level that are of profound significance to physiotherapists'.

Bone tapping

Light sharp taps on bony points can be used to facilitate movement towards the point tapped if used on the same sclerotome as the mytome of muscle to be facilitated.

Example (i) Tap on the dorsal aspect of the radial styloid to facilitate radial wrist extension and inhibit ulnar flexion.

Example (ii) Tap on the anterior aspect of the lateral maleolus to facilitate eversion and dorsiflexion and inhibit plantar-flexion and inversion.

Position of head in space and in relation to the rest of body

Choice of position of the head in space and in relation to the trunk is carefully made in consideration to the input from the labyrinth of the inner ear and to input from facet joints of the neck. In adults with hemiplegia, the tonic labyrinth or tonic neck reflexes may be released and influence spasticity on the affected side. Tonic laby-rinthine reflex activity increases extensor tone in supine, reduces it in prone and reduces extensor tone on the uppermost side in side lying. Side lying on the unaffected side is selected so that anti-gravity and extensor thrust patterns of spasticity are reduced. The extensor thrust of the leg is often a feature of stroke patients and the retraction of shoulder girdle and typical position of shoulder, elbow and wrist and hand appear to be antigravity postures of an upper limb used to cling to a tree or parent primate. Both patterns are primitive synergies modified, as the neuromuscular system develops, to allow prehension of upper limb and weight bearing on the lower limb. Prone lying will also inhibit spasticity in extensors and shoulder retractors. Burke (1980) speculates that input from neck and labyrinth produces reflexes with alternative control mech-anism for fast and slow muscles.

In all cases, even where there is no evidence of abnormal tonic reflexes, input from labyrinth and from vertebral joints is recruited. Careful selection of total body position and alignment of head and trunk facilitates correct posture even if perceptual defects or other sensory loss is present.

The principle is to consider the whole body position, select stimuli and sequences of activity so as to elicit good function. Successful regimes are repeated and ways found for the patient or relatives to repeat simple methods of achieving basic activities.

ASSESSMENT

A survey is made of all factors contributing to dysfunction and to domestic environment so that needs are identified. Rood's approach is to look for syndromes of sensory and perceptual defects and patterns of motor disability. It is essential to recognise how motor activity is blocked or distorted by non-use of existing nerve path-ways. Also considered is the imbalance in sensitivity to stretch in groups of muscles and their antagonists.

As discussed above, stimuli are selected and sequences of activities chosen to correct the observed imbalance. Some examples of the selection of stimuli will be indicated. Included are observation and testing of skilled use of limbs.

The level of independence is found in communication, manipulative skills for self-care and gross motor functions of changes in position, transfers and locomotion. Mental and emotional problems must be identified and conference with the clinical psychologist sought if necessary. Certain points relevant to selection of stimuli and techniques used in treatment will be discussed but not details of clinical examination.

Sensation and perception. Defective sensation and perception must be identified but their presence does not reduce the pertinence of stimulation of receptors in skin and deep dermis, joints or bone: indeed, it makes their use essential. The lesions producing hemiplegia are cephaloid to centres in brain-stem, cerebellum and spinal cord, so nerve impulses reaching such intact centres can produce an effect. If repeated over a sufficient period of time, stimuli may have a beneficial trophic influence on the C.N.S. The patient may regain awareness of the affected side which will facilitate its use. Writing of so-called 'body image' defect Williams (1979) states; 'The patient is carrying around, as it were, a phantom of himself, and in the absence of severe or prolonged external stimulation, lives with this phantom instead of with reality'. Prolonged external stimulation can be provided as described in the section on stimuli and is thus beneficial in ameliorating these states.

Observation of motor abilities. Absence or abnormality of postural reactions, quality of voluntary movement, muscle tone and predominant patterns of spasticity must be noted. Release of tonic neck or labyrinthine reflexes elicited by testing or observed during spontaneous movement by the patient, should be recognised. The presence of a grasp reflex in hand or foot must be considered.

A clinical method of grading the severity of spasticity and its effect on quality of movement is described by Goff (1976). Its use assists treatment planning and particularly evaluation.

A method of reducing the grasp reflex is described in the appendix as is the technique used for spasticity in unarthrodial muscles in contrast to that used for multiarthrodial muscles, mainly flexors and adductors. The different characteristics of flexor withdrawal and extensor thrust reflexes necessitates the selection of one or other techniques described. Flexion withdrawal, involving mainly quick acting motor units in multiarthrodial muscles, is a transient reflex resulting in removal of the end of a limb from a potentially harmful stimulus. The spinal reflex arc is multi-segmental ipsilateral and, unless the stimulus is repeated or hyper-sensitive flexors are stretched by the force of gravity as they relax, the response is transient. In contrast, the extensor thrust of a leg persists when it is part of a crossed extensor reflex or in response to pressure on the ball of the foot. It also persists as part of a total extension reflex of head, trunk and legs. If resistance is given to a limb in an extensor reflex pattern it may exhibit the 'clasp knife' or lengthening reaction of suddenly relaxing. Slow stretch is thus effective in reducing tone in slow-acting motor units of uniarthro-dial muscles, but resistance or stretch to quick-acting motor units in multiarthrodial muscles increases their hypertonicity so must be avoided. Contrasting characteristics of spinal flexor and extensor reflexes are summarised by Bell et al (1954).

Apraxis. This disability is very perplexing for patients and rela-tives who do not understand the reason for it. Moreover, the harder the patient concentrates on performing a task the less likely is he to succeed, By persistent repetition of automatically induced use of the part, pathways may be re-established or new ones utilised so that better function results. Neurology of apraxis and the forms it takes is discussed by Williams (1979).

CONCLUSION

The clinical state of each patient may fluctuate as well as change with the passage of time. The therapist must be observant, sensitive to changes of mood as well as of clinical states and, most import-antly, must evaluate the effectiveness of treatment. Ways should be devised to show patients and relatives how to apply successful stimulation and facilitation so that good function is maintained and further professional treatment unnecessary.

A selection of ideas used in the treatment of stroke will be discussed in an appendix. Those selected are inspired by Rood's concept of the application of neuro-physiology to physical therapy. Research is proceeding into explanations of how afferent infor-mation from receptors within and on the surface of the body is integrated. It is now understood that although neurons are not replaced if lost through pathological states, changes at molecular level can change the form and function of both neurons and muscle tissue. This offers physiotherapists an exciting challenge since it is by persistent repetition of regimes of activity that these trophic influences may eventually produce changes in form and allow better function.

APPENDIX

Descriptions will be given of sequences and stimuli at various stages and will relate to clinical states as discussed in the section on assessment. Combinations of signs and symptoms will be different for each individual as will the severity of these. Response to treatment also varies, so it is essential that the treatment programme is modified according to the needs of each patient as their clinical state changes. No set routine can be stated but a broad outline of suggestions is given for various syndromes.

EARLY STAGES OF HYPO-TONE AND LACK OF POSTURAL REACTIONS

The following techniques aim to elicit normal muscle tone and to prevent spasticity, or at least to avoid reinforcement of spasticity. Postural reactions are used for basic motor activities.

Starting positions: patient lying or side lying

Stimuli used

The therapist should:
1. Brush all areas to increase fusimotor inflow to muscles required for stability and basic movements and to inhibit fusimotor inflow to their antagonists.
2. Brush especially the area(s) of skin with the same nerve root supply and on the same surface as those muscles likely to be opposed by strong spastic antagonists when muscle tone increases. For example:

   a. Arm: brush skin over dorsal interossei, thenar and hypothenar areas, radial side of extensor aspect of forearm, medial head of triceps, anterior fibres of deltoid and clavicular fibres of pectoralis major. (See Figures 5.1a and b).
   b. Leg: brush skin on dorsum of foot between toes, skin over extensor digitorum and peronei, over the insertion of sartorius and up along the belly of this muscle.
   c. Brush lateral side of thigh *opposite* adductors of hip but with the same root supply so inhibiting fusimotor inflow to adductors.

Activities using total movement patterns

The therapist should:
(i) Facilitate rolling to both sides.
(ii) Total flexion: head, trunk limbs. Omit total extension.

Starting position: crook lying

The therapist should:
(i) Place and hold affected leg in correct position.
(ii) Place affected arm across chest.

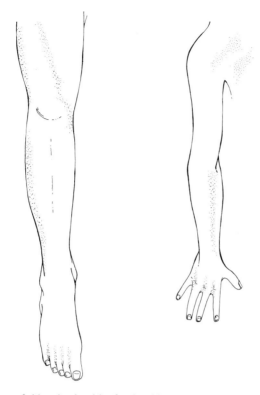

Fig. 5.1   Areas of skin stimulated by fast brushing.

(iii) Place a small pad under the occiput to tilt the skull and reduce any cervical lordosis. The neck should be flat and the chin tucked in.

Stimuli

(i) With the head and neck in a symmetrical position and neither flexed nor extended pressure is given from the top of the head down towards the trunk to activate cocontraction of deep postural muscles of the neck and trunk.

(ii) Pressure is given down from knee to heel and up through the long axis of the femur to the hip joint. This is maintained whilst ensuring a good position of the affected leg, i.e. the foot should be flat on the supporting surface and the hip neither medially nor laterally rotated and in slight abduction. This should elicit cocontraction of deep proximal muscles and enable the patient to maintain the crook position unaided.

(iii) The forearm is rubbed firmly over the posterior border of the ulna (see Fig. 5.2). Pressure is applied from the ulnar side of the heel of the hand, i.e. from pisiform up through the forearm (see Fig. 5.3). Pressure is applied from below the elbow up through the long axis of the humerus. The position of the head of humerus in relation to the glenoid cavity of the scapula must be correct

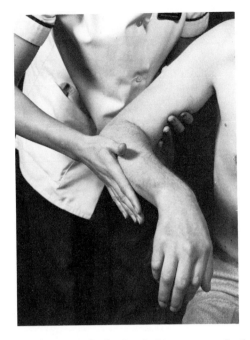

Fig. 5.2 Firm rub along posterior border of ulnar to prepare for forearm support.

for weight bearing on an arm and can be maintained in a good position by the therapist whilst giving counter pressure to the compressing force applied from below the elbow (see Fig. 5.4).

Activities using support of body weight over fixed distal segments and movements over this

(i) Bridging: the therapist should assist if necessary to ensure good position of affected leg by holding the foot, and facilitate by (a) pressure from knee to foot and knee to hip, and (b) bone tap over anterior iliac spine in the direction of required movement to raise the pelvis on the affected side. The patient should then progress to moving the pelvis, once lifted, to alternate sides, and to half-crook lying with the unaffected leg extended, pelvic lifting with only the affected leg fixed distally.

(ii) With pressure and support under the forearm by the therapist's hands to emulate a weight-bearing position, the patient is instructed to push the elbow forwards. This should gain stability at shoulder girdle and shoulder and prepare for weight bearing.

Starting position: side lying on unaffected side

The head is supported so that it is in a neutral symmetrical position. The unaffected limb is flexed at hip and knee. The top (affected) leg is either with flexion and

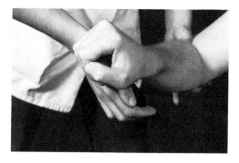

Fig. 5.3 Pressure on heel of hand ulnar side and counter-pressure from behind elbow along axis of forearm to gain stability of wrist joint; note wrist held in radial extension.

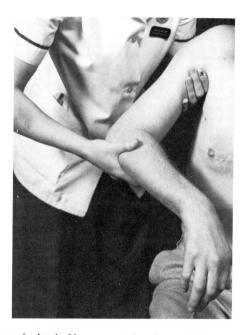

Fig. 5.4 Support for head of humerus at gleno-humeral joint, pressure given up through humerus to elicit stability and muscular control proximally.

adduction at hip and flexion at knee, or with extension and some abduction at hip and with knee flexed. These positions discourage total spastic synergies of the leg. The top arm (affected limb) is placed in forearm support position in front of the patient.

Stimuli

 (i) Brushing areas of arm as previously described may be repeated.
(ii) Pressure is applied from shoulder to elbow and down on the forearm to the posterior border of the ulnar. The weight of the body must be taken by the therapist until it is felt that the deep muscles of shoulder girdle and shoulder are stabilising the position.

Activity

The therapist should encourage the patient to:
 (i) Rock over the supporting, affected forearm, rolling the upper trunk forward and backward. Assistance to keep a correct position may be needed.
(ii) Progress to side sitting supporting the trunk with affected arm. Assistance may be needed to stabilise the extended elbow and to support some of the body weight until the patient's muscles work to stabilise the position.

Starting position: supported sitting in a chair

The head and trunk must be symmetrical and the back straight, the legs placed so that hips and knees are at 90° of flexion with both feet flat on the floor; the hips must be slightly abducted and in neutral rotation.

Stimuli

  (i) Pressure is given through the head and trunk and down on affected shoulder until a symmetrical head and trunk posture is maintained unaided.
 (ii) Pressure is given from knee to hip and knee to heel until the correct leg position is maintained unaided.
(iii) Arm stimuli are repeated as in lying.

Activities

The patient should:
  (i) Push and reach forward with both arms, facilitated by bi-lateral movement and pressure on heel of affected hand by the therapist who should assist if required.
 (ii) Reach across trunk with affected hand towards opposite shoulder; facilitate by pushing unaffected hand which offers resistance. The patient can be shown how to assist the movement whilst giving pressure to the affected hand (see Fig. 5.5).
(iii) Press affected elbow down into palm of unaffected hand which gives resistance; lift affected hand to mouth actively.
 (iv) Lean forwards and backwards and from side to side keeping heels down and feet firmly fixed on the floor.
  (v) Progress to lifting the buttocks off the chair as in preparing to stand up. All activities should be repeated many times at one session.

A problem may arise through lack of balance reactions, the patient falling towards the affected side. To increase sensitivity to stretch in the deep back muscles, especially those on the unaffected side, a pillow is placed on the arm of the chair on the affected side and the patient is positioned so that he leans sideways over the pillow: that is, the tendency to fall to the side is not corrected but increased. Usually the response to this is automatic straightening of the back. Self-correction is thus obtained and can be further facilitated and maintained by firm pressure downwards

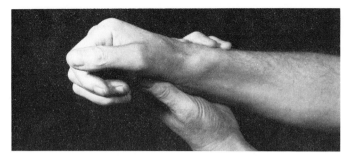

Fig. 5.5   Patients unaffected left hand is facilitating reaching forward with affected right hand by giving pressure with his left thumb to region of right pisiform; his fingers and hand at the same time can assist the stretching reaching movement of the affected arm.

on the shoulders, the lower shoulder being given most pressure so that the patient straightens automatically.

Starting position: forearm support stoop sitting

The positions of the head, trunk and legs are corrected as in sitting and arms are placed on a table of suitable height in front of the patient.

Stimuli

The therapist should apply pressure on shoulder and forearm, which must be in correct alignment for weight bearing.

Activity moving over a fixed distal segment

The patient should:
  (i) Move from side to side and forwards and backwards, keeping both arms and both feet firmly on the support of the table and floor. The trunk rocks from side to side, or forwards and backwards.
 (ii) Lift buttocks off the chair a few inches. Repeat frequently.
(iii) Take affected hand to mouth keeping the elbow on the table. (In suitable cases the patient can be shown how to give facilitation to the affected arm by pressing down on the forearm with the other hand.) Progress to rising to supported standing when possible.

Starting position: standing. Support if required by therapist on the affected side

Stimuli

The therapist should apply compression from hip to knee whilst ensuring that the hip is well forward and that the knee is not hyperextended. The affected arm is extended at elbow and pressure is given from heel of hand to shoulder.

Activities moving over fixed distal segments and progressing to movement with distal end free

The patient should:
(i) Shift weight backwards, forwards and sideways.
(ii) With weight on affected leg, step forwards and backwards with unaffected leg. Correct swing through pattern must be stressed. The patient's attention is directed to the ease of leg movement during the swing phase of walking. As the leg steps forward movement occurs freely at the hip and as the knee straightens heel strike occurs and the forefoot clears the floor. Small ranges of movement of the unaffected leg should prevent collapse or thrust of the affected leg. Repeat many times in correct sequence of movement.
(iii) Repeat (ii) with alternate leg. Assistance may be needed to ensure a correct pattern of swing through with affected leg.
(iv) Walk, taking small steps and assisted and facilitated by the therapist.
(v) Practise sitting from standing, standing from sitting, making sure the weight is taken on both legs equally and that the weight of the trunk is well forward with shoulders above the knees. The arms should be extended in front of the patient and the head should lead by ensuring that the patient looks up and forward as he stands up.
(vi) Practice transfers, chair to bed, etc.

Length of treatment sessions

Many short periods of stimulation and activity daily are ideal in the early stages and all personnel concerned with the care of the patient should be shown the best way to elicit good posture and how to facilitate transfers.

Rate of progress will vary and ideally the patient should not be expected to attempt transfers or gait until good posture and balance reactions are re-established.

Other positions which can be used for treatment and activities

These should include prone lying, forearm support prone lying, forearm support prone kneeling and prone kneeling. In all these, weight should not be taken on the affected arm or leg, unless it is in correct alignment. Assistance and facilitation are given as required. When stability is sufficient to allow the patient to hold the position unaided, activities are progressed by rocking over fixed distal parts and finally to basic activities moving the distal end of the arm and leg. Examples of the latter are crawling, taking hand to mouth or reaching for objects and moving from one position to another (see Fig. 5.6).

Other problems

Problems such as poor circulation to the hand or foot, lack of sensation and perception, will be reduced by fast brushing to all surfaces of the hand, forearm, foot and leg. The patient is instructed to rub the affected side lightly with the fingertips of the other hand frequently throughout the day. During treatment sessions the therapist constantly provides feedback to the patient about the position or activity of the affected side as it is moved or positioned. As the hand is brought towards the opposite side of the body the therapist should say 'feel your hand with your shoulder, or feel your hand with your face'. In this way the patient is made aware of the affected side.

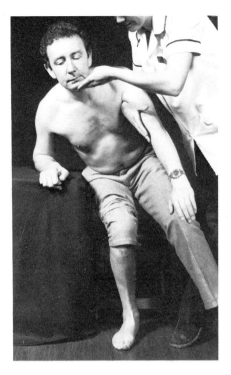

Fig. 5.6 Patient prepares to rise to standing not using unaffected side; therapist reminds him to keep the head up and gives minimal support on unaffected side.

Treatment if muscle tone is increased i.e. spastic type

The increase of muscle tone in some cases after a stroke may occur rapidly; in others it increases very gradually. In a minority of cases with residual loss of sensation or perception, a state of hypotone persists. In the majority of cases, however, muscle tone returns and is increased, presenting as spasticity. Spastic synergic movements prevent good function unless treatment successfully reduces the abnormal hypertone and restores postural reactions. Other expressions of release symptoms are a grasp reflex and an exaggerated flexor withdrawal reflex of the affected leg.

Grasp reflex

Slow firm massage to the centre of the palm of hand distal to the weight-bearing area on the proximal part is given for several minutes avoiding stretch of the long finger flexors or contact with the finger tips. This technique appears to desensitise the hand and is repeated at each treatment session until it is no longer needed. The massage is given after brushing as described above and is followed by techniques to encourage weight-bearing on the hand.

Hyperactive flexor withdrawal of leg

This problem sometimes occurs in very frail patients too ill to sit out of bed. Relief usually follows if two or three minutes of firm massage is given to the sole of the foot in the non-weight-bearing areas of the instep. Firm pressure on the plantar surface of the heel is then given and pressure from heel to knee and knee to hip prepares for weight-bearing in crook lying. Activities are elicited and assisted, such as pelvic lifting, moving across or up and down the bed.

Grasp reflex of the foot

If this occurs a similar regime of treatment is used as for flexor withdrawal of the leg.

SPASTICITY OF THE UPPER LIMB

At each treatment the position and activity of the whole body is considered, but for clarity some techniques used for specific regions will be discussed separately.

Starting position: side lying on unaffected side

The whole body should be positioned carefully as described above. Gentle rocking of the pelvis may be needed to reduce spasticity in the trunk and leg before the leg can be placed correctly.

Stimuli

The therapist should:
  (i) Brush areas of skin as previously described.
 (ii) Slowly stretch the retractors of the shoulder girdle and posterior deltoid muscle. The arm is gradually brought across the front of the chest and held there for at least five minutes. The patient may be able to hold this position with the unaffected arm, so releasing the therapist's hands for treatment of the hand or leg. An added benefit, if the patient can help in this way, is that he is made aware of the affected arm and its position in relation to the body.
(iii) Place a firm cone-shaped object, such as a cardboard or plastic spool used in the weaving trade, in the hand with the larger open end towards the little finger. Apply pressure on the back of the hand so as to mould gradually the hand around the cone (see Figs. 5.7a, b and 5.8). The pressure over the distal attachments of flexor superficialis digitorum and on the palmar surface of the metacarpals reflexly reduces spasticity in the flexors and adductors of the fingers and the fingertips gradually relax. The thumb is gradually pressed around the cone and brought into a position of abduction in a plane at right angles to the hand. It is gradually rotated so that the palmar surface is in contact with the cone. The pressure on the hand holding the cone should be maintained until a good position of the hand is retained without pressure. The patient is asked to try to hold the cone without grasping it with the thumb and fingertips. The cone can be turned in the patient's hand to increase awareness of skin sensation. As this is done by the therapist, it must be observed whether a grasp reflex is elicited. Should this occur, firm massage is applied to the palm. As the cone is retained in the hand, pressure is given, by the therapist, through the open end of the cone up through the ulnar side of the heel of the hand through the

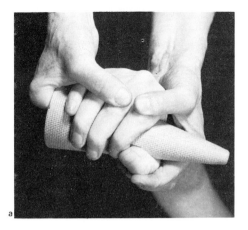

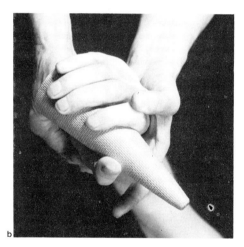

Fig. 5.7a and b Cone placed in hand wide end towards 5th digit. Therapist's right hand gives pressure from inside of cone to pisiform, i.e. ulnar side of heel of hand; left hand moulds hand around cone giving pressure over D.I.P. joint of index to gain release of digitorum superficialis.

forearm and arm. Deep postural muscles of the whole arm are facilitated in this way and spasticity is reduced.

(iv) Non-resisted repeated small range movements of elbow, wrist and fingers without facilitation are used to reduce spasticity in the flexors. Patients find this technique difficult to learn, and need to concentrate, but must not be given any assistance or any form of facilitation. This procedure can be used before use of a cone or can be done with the cone held by the patient. Combination of techniques described will summate the effect of each and the arm should now be ready for activities.

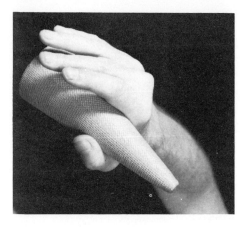

Fig. 5.8   Patient can now hold cone without palmar grip with finger tips.

Activities preparing for good arm function

Activities include weight bearing on the forearms or hand, reaching, pushing, taking an object towards the mouth or above the head. These are encouraged by appropriate stimuli such as pressure on the heel of the hand as the patient is asked to push gently. The sequences used follow the basic principle of using the part in total movement patterns; then for support, progressing to movement over the supporting forearm or hand and finally free skilled use of the hand (see Figs. 5.9, 5.10 and 5.11).

Any convenient starting position can be used for the techniques described for reduction of spasticity, and followed by activities which are of immediate use to the patient. For example, a patient may sit with both arms on a table, practise reaching forward with both hands and, finally, bring it to the mouth as if drinking.

SPASTICITY OF THE LEG

Starting positions

These are crook lying, prone lying, with affected knee flexed, and lying.

Stimuli

(i) Brushing as above.
(ii) Slow maintained stretch to soleus everting the foot as it is dorsiflexed, thus stretching the medial part of the soleus. The therapist should avoid sudden pressure on the ball of foot but pull the heel down gradually and as the calf relaxes use the forearm to give added leverage along the sole of the foot. The patient is asked to try to pull the foot up and out. Stretch should be maintained on the full length of soleus for at least five minutes, whilst the knee remains flexed. As reduction of spasticity occurs the position can usually be held by one

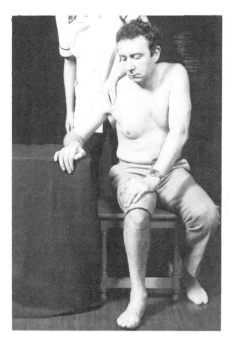

Fig. 5.9 Patient takes weight through affected forearm. Therapist puts weight down through humerus to elbow and forearm to prepare for using right arm and leg for support and to rise to standing without using unaffected arm or leg. His left arm gives pressure down from right knee to heel.

      hand, the other can then give firm pressure from the plantar surface of medial side of the heel up through the leg.

(iii) The therapist should tap lightly the lateral malleolus to facilitate eversion and dorsiflexion.

(iv) Repeated small range non-resisted movements of adduction of hip are taught and repeated many times without facilitation. In teaching this it is necessary to ensure that the adductors are used and that the movement is not just a rolling in and out but true adduction and abduction. Stimulation is then given by resistance and a brisk command to 'abduct widely'. The whole technique is repeated starting with a greater degree of abduction. This technique can be used with knees flexed as in crook lying or with knees extended. In the latter case friction is reduced by supporting the heels by the therapist's hands. The therapist must not, however, assist or resist the volitional movements. A simple check with a tape measure to show that range has increased and that adductors have relaxed encourages both patient and therapist.

    As with the arm, the benefit of each technique is summated and the leg is now ready for activities including bridging, transfers and gait.

Starting position: sitting

Good symmetrical posture must be obtained as described for the early stage.

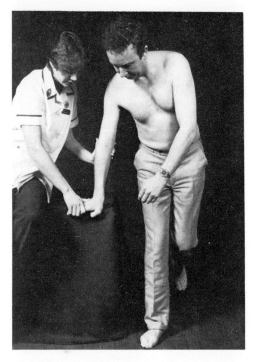

Fig. 5.10 Patient stands with weight through an extended right arm and weight correctly taken on right leg.

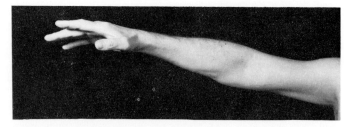

Fig. 5.11 Following the above sequences the patient is able to maintain a good position of right arm and hand.

Stimuli

(i) Brushing dorsum of foot, over extensor digitorum and peronei and on lateral side of thigh.

(ii) Slow stretch of soleus by pressure down from the knee to the heel. The patient is helped to move gradually the thigh and trunk forward over the affected leg whilst keeping the heel on the floor. In this way dorsi-flexion is increased and soleus slowly lengthened. The foot is then brought back, increasing flexion at the knee and dorsi-flexion at the ankle. Pressure is given at the knee to retain the heel position in contact with the floor. Greater pressure is exerted down towards the medial side of the heel than to the lateral side to inhibit inversion of foot. If possible the patient is taught to control the position of the affected leg by use of the unaffected hand (see Fig. 5.9). When a good position of the leg is obtained the patient can place the affected hand on his knee, cover this with the unaffected hand and give pressure through both the heel of the affected hand and affected leg (see Fig. 5.12). The position is maintained for at least five minutes.

(iii) Non-resisted small range movements of adduction and abduction at hip are repeated many times and followed by facilitation to gain abduction.

Activities

The patient should:
(i) Practise active eversion with dorsi-flexion firstly on the unaffected side, then bilaterally and finally alternately. The heels remain on the floor and extension of the big toe is discouraged. On the affected side pressure down by the therapist on the medial side of the heel and light tapping on the lateral malleolus facilitates the response.

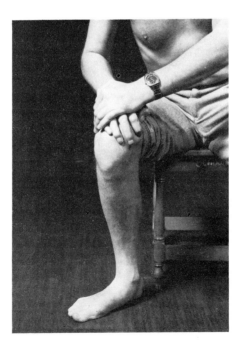

Fig. 5.12 Patient having gained inhibition of tone in soleus by a slow stretch in sitting, gives pressure down through knee to heel; his left hand is simultaneously giving pressure to heel on right hand and right leg to inhibit spasticity in both.

 (ii) Taking weight on the heels, shift the buttocks from side to side.
(iii) Lean well forward with both arms reaching forwards and upwards; look upwards and ahead and start to extend knees, raising the buttocks off the chair. The knees are not fully extended and weight is taken equally on both heels. The movement is slow and controlled and is followed by an equally controlled sitting down. The patient is encouraged to practise this many times and repeat frequently the regime for reducing tone. If the patient is sitting on the side of a high mat he can practise moving sideways without using his unaffected arm. Movement should be towards his affected side.
(iv) Stand from sitting, and weight transfer and step as described for the early stage.
 (v) Negotiate slopes, curbs, steps and stairs safely. The affected leg should lead up steps and the unaffected one lead down. Good control is needed for this and each individual's ability must be assessed before the therapist chooses the pattern of stair climbing which is to be taught.

It is important to form associations with the patient's environment whilst practising functional activities. All personnel concerned with his care should try to use the same methods of instruction or assistance as those used in treatment sessions. Ideally, treatment should also be given in the ward or in the patient's own home.

SPASTICITY OF TRUNK AND NECK

Starting position: modified crook lying

Stimuli

The therapist should:
 (i) Brush skin over the front of the neck and over rectus abdominus, thus reducing the sensitivity to stretch in deep posterior neck and trunk muscles.
(ii) Give slow stretch to deep posterior neck and trunk muscles. This is achieved by tilting the head so that the chin is tucked in, the neck flat and the external occipital protuberance rotates upwards away from the spine. A small pad or wedge under the occiput maintains the position. The pelvis is rotated or tilted so that the lumbar spine is flat and the anterior superior iliac spines are rotated up towards the thorax. The position is maintained by placing a wedge under the buttocks. The wedge is only a few inches deep at its deepest side which is towards the feet. The legs are in a crook-lying position and the arms crossed in front of the body. The position is maintained for five minutes at least.

Symmetrical head position is essential and can be facilitated by pressure down from the top of the head and through the spine. The position can be used while the arm and leg are treated.

Activities

Whilst maintaining a good head and trunk posture, bilateral arm and leg movements are practised. Progression to sitting and standing with good posture follows correction in crook lying.

TREATMENT FOR HYPOTONE OF FACIAL MUSCLES

In the early stages the lower part of the face lacks tone on the affected side. Patients are very distressed by the resulting dysarthria and difficulty in swallowing.

Starting position

Any convenient position can be used so long as the head is symmetrical and in neutral position.

Stimuli

The therapist should:
(i) Brush lightly around the lips starting on the unaffected side and avoiding contact below the lower lip. Repeat two or three times. Brush with light quick strokes up and out from the corner of the mouth. Start on the unaffected side two or three strokes then repeat on affected side.
(ii) Touch the lips lightly with an ice cube or ice-lollipop.

Activities

(i) The patient is told to pucker the lips and make sucking actions. Resistance is given by finger tips applied to the unaffected side and to the affected side if the muscles on that side are working.
(ii) The patient then sucks up through a straw cold, unsweetened fruit juice. The straw can be placed against an ice cube in the drink and the patient sucks through it. This gives resistance to the sucking, so facilitating the action and also eliciting swallowing. This results in melting a hole in the ice cube and so fun and motivation become added facilitations.
(iii) Swallowing is facilitated by brief applications of ice to the front of the neck, just above the suprasternal notch. A firm stroke downwards on the larynx will also elicit swallowing. For all feeding, chewing food, swallowing solids and liquids, a good position of head and trunk should be used with the trunk and head vertical but so that a little flexion is needed to take the food or drink into the mouth.

ACKNOWLEDGEMENTS

Many thanks to staff in the Medical Photography Department and to the secretarial staff of the School of Physiotherapy, Robert Jones and Agnes Hunt Orthopaedic Hospital, Oswestry.

REFERENCES

Bell G H, Davidson J N Scarborough M, 1954 The pathways of the spinal cord. In: Textbook of physiology and biochemistry. E.S. Livingston, Edinburgh, ch 46, p 787

Bethune D B 1975 Neurophysiological facilitation of respiration in the unconscious adult patient. Physiotherapy Canada 27(5): 241–245

Boyd I A 1980 The action of the three types of intrafusal muscle. In: Taylor, Prochazka (eds) Muscle receptors and movement. MacMillan, London, p 17

Burke R E 1980 Motor unit types. Trends in Neuroscience 3(11): 255–258. Elsevier, North Holland

Goff B 1969 Excitatory cold. Physiotherapy 55(11): 467–468

Goff B 1972 The application of recent advances in neurophysiology to Miss Rood's concept of neuromuscular facilitation. Physiotherapy 58(12): 409–415

Goff B 1976 Grading of spasticity and its effect on voluntary movement. Physiotherapy 62(11): 358–361

Haase J, Cleveland S, Ross H G 1975 Problems of postsynaptic autogenous recurrent inhibition in mammalian spinal cord. Reviews of Physiology, Biochemistry and Pharmacology 73: 73–129

Hunt C C, Perl E R 1960 Spindle reflex mechanisms concerned with skeletal muscle. Physiological Reviews 40: 538–579

Kidd G (1980) Neuro-muscular control of the skeleton. In: Owen R, Goodfellow J, Bullough P (eds) Scientific foundations of orthopaedics and traumatology. Heinemann, London, ch 17, p 115–125

Kidd G (1983) Personal communication, Lecture notes

Kidd G, Brodie P 1980 The motor unit. A review. Physiotherapy 66(5): 146–152

Loeb G E, Hoffer J A 1980 Muscle spindle function. In: Taylor, Prochazka (eds) Muscle receptors and movement. Macmillan, London, p 129

Matthews P B C 1973 The advances of the last decade of animal experimentation upon muscle spindles. The background to current human work. In: Desmedt J E (ed) New developments in electromyography and clinical neurology, vol 3. Skarger, Basel, p 95–97

Rood M S 1956 Neurophysiological mechanisms utilised in the treatment of neuromuscular dysfunction. American Journal of Occupational Therapy 4(II): 220–225

Tracey D J 1980 Joint receptors and the control of movement. Trends in Neuroscience. 3(11): 211–226

Vallbo A B, Hagbarth K E, Torebjork H E, Wallin B G 1979 Somatosensory proprioceptive and sympathetic activity in human peripheral nerves. Physiological Reviews 59(5):919

Williams M 1979 Disorders of bodily awareness. In: Brain damage, behaviour and the mind. John Wiley & Son, Chichester, ch 6, p 78–87

Williams M 1979 Dirorders of motor skill. In: Brain damage, behaviour and the mind. John Wiley & Son, Chichester, ch 7, p 88–96

Wyke B D 1972 Articular neurology. A Review. Physiotherapy 53(3): 94–99

Biofeedback in the treatment of hemiplegia

INTRODUCTION

The concept of feedback is fundamental to the maintenance of homeostasis in man. Physiological events such as blood pressure, endocrine secretion and body temperature are regulated by negative feedback from sensitive devices which continuously monitor these functions. Normal movement is controlled by a complex feedback system. This is most clearly seen in the acquisition of a new skill such as the throwing of a dart. The target on the darts board is defined visually and a dart is thrown by a rapid movement of the arm as dictated by a sequence of motor impulses from the central nervous system. Information regarding the force and timing of the movement is received from muscle and joint proprioceptors while the placement of the dart is noted visually. The desired and actual achievements are compared and modifications are made to subsequent movements based upon the interaction of these two senses (Fig. 6.1 input a & b).

Biofeedback may be defined as the creation of a new feedback loop between the periphery and the brain to aid in self-regulation (Fig. 6.1 input c). The word is synonymous with the term 'biological feedback'. It denotes a method of obtaining accurate and instantaneous information from certain biological events which are usually regulated without conscious control. It normally involves the use of electronic equipment which will monitor and amplify the physiological signals and reveal them in forms which are easily understood and interpreted by the subject. Biofeedback therapy is based upon the assumption that voluntary control can be increased with an increase in relevant afferent information. When this is presented in the auditory and visual displays of biofeedback, the subject can learn to affect consciously the signals by imposing some degree of volition upon the events producing them. In this way, subjects have been trained to modify physiological parameters such as muscle

BODY

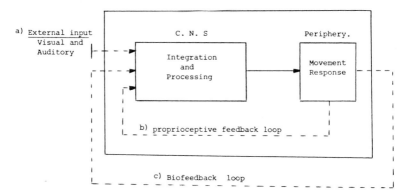

Fig. 6.1 Diagrammatic representation of normal exteroceptive and proprioceptive feedback to the Central Nervous System, with additional biofeedback loop.

tone, heart rate, blood pressure and skin temperature over selected areas, such as the hands. When applied clinically, this can give patients a measure of control over tension and migraine headaches (Sargent et al, 1972), hypertension (Kristt & Engel, 1975), and over psychosomatic disorders such as asthma (Kotses et al, 1977). The most promising area of application, however, is undoubtedly that of neuromuscular re-education. EMG biofeedback has been successfully used in the treatment of poliomyelitis (Marinacci & Horande, 1960), peripheral nerve damage (Brown et al, 1978) and in the rehabilitation of neurological conditions, especially hemiplegia. Selected studies in this area will be examined in more detail.

EMG BIOFEEDBACK IN STROKE REHABILITATION— REVIEW OF STUDIES

Reports of successful applications of biofeedback in the treatment of hemiplegia over the past 25 years have stimulated considerable interest among physiotherapists and other health professionals. Yet physiotherapists on the whole have been slow to incorporate biofeedback into the normal treatment regimes for stroke patients. One reason for this may be a reluctance to accept that the improvement claimed by many authors could be attributed solely to biofeedback. Factors such as motivation and spontaneous recovery which are known to make a significant contribution towards the eventual outcome in all neurological rehabilitation make the evaluation of any form of treatment difficult. Over the past decade, however, a number of controlled studies which have sought to eliminate all possible variables from biofeedback research have supported the earlier claims for this form of therapy. These cannot be dismissed lightly. Much can be learned from a consideration of all forms of biofeedback research, but only a limited number can be included here. The studies reviewed in this chapter have been selected to demonstrate a range of factors such as variations in research design and measurement of outcome. For purposes of clarity they will be considered in relation to anatomical location.

The upper limb

The first recorded use of EMG biofeedback in the treatment of the upper limb was that of Marinacci and Horande (1960) of a 64-year-old man suffering from left-sided hemiplegia as a result of thrombosis of the middle cerebral artery. Following a demonstration of biofeedback using the deltoid muscle of the unaffected side, the electrodes were transferred to the affected shoulder and the patient was able to activate from 10% to 15% of the motor units in the previously inactive deltoid muscle. This procedure was repeated in the triceps brachii and in the flexor and extensor muscles of the wrist. Within an hour the patient was able to develop approximately 20% of function in the muscles of the left arm. The importance of this report is now widely recognised, yet with the exception of a few isolated studies (e.g. Andrews, 1964) almost a decade was to pass before serious research into the value of EMG biofeedback was established.

EMG biofeedback training has been focused upon all the major muscle groups of the upper limb and their associated movements. Success in counteracting subluxation of the shoulder was reported in a study involving 13 patients carried out by Basmajian and associates. Emphasis during training was placed upon improving scapular mobility and the restoration of proper orientation of the glenoid cavity by re-educating the trapezius and the deltoid muscles. Radiographic assessment demonstrated improvement in almost all subjects (Basmajian et al, 1977). A controlled study carried out by Skelly and Kenedi (1982) on 20 stroke patients was designed to increase control of flexion of the shoulder joint. The anterior fibres of the deltoid were selected for re-education purposes. An increase in function was obtained in 45% of patients in the experimental group (patients with sensory loss), and in 77% of patients in the control group (patients with normal sensation). While in some subjects this improvement was limited to an increase in muscle tension, several achieved active elevation of the arm from the dependent to the horizontal position through an arc of 90 degrees. Both of these studies indicate an increase in shoulder function attributed to biofeedback therapy. A different outcome emerged from an investigation undertaken by Lee and co-workers. In their research, patients were encouraged to contract the deltoid muscle isometrically for a period of 5 seconds, followed by a relaxation phase lasting 10 seconds. This was repeated continuously for 5 minutes allowing a total of 20 contractions. Training was carried out on three successive days under three experimental conditions, viz. true myofeedback, placebo myofeedback (when the electrical activity from a muscle of the examiner's arm was relayed to the feedback device), and therapeutic exercise without feedback. The integral EMG was the parameter chosen for evaluation purposes. When analysed, the results for true myofeedback paralleled those obtained during therapeutic exercise, but all patients showed regression under placebo conditions. It was concluded that EMG biofeedback has a non-specific effect in its short term application (Lee et al, 1976). This study was later criticised by Middaugh & Millar (1980) who demonstrated that a minimum of 10 seconds is required before the integral EMG is likely to reach its peak value under biofeedback conditions.

Success in training the movements of the elbow joint has been claimed in relation to the re-activation of paretic muscles (Andrews, 1964) and also in the inhibition of spasticity in the biceps (Kleinman et al, 1976). In both studies, patients acquired not only an increase in muscle function but also a greater active range of movement.

Selective movements of the wrist and hand are seldom regained following hemiplegia, and re-education using biofeedback has on the whole yielded disappointing results. The dominance of patho-logical synergies presents a major obstacle to the restoration of hand function. Attempts to break up such synergies using biofeedback have included the re-training of the wrist extensor muscles in their role as prime movers and then as synergists when making a first (Nafpliotis, 1976); also the simultaneous monitoring of agonists and antagonists (Prevo et al, 1982). A second problem involves the transfer of recently acquired ability into functional use of the hand. In a research programme undertaken by Brudny et al (1976) func-tion graded as 'assistive capacity' and 'prehension' was established in more than 60% of patients, but it was later noted that many did not in fact use their hand in activities of daily living. Similar findings were obtained by Wolf and associates in relation to 48 patients of whom it was noted, 'while appreciable gains in control of elbow and shoulder function could be achieved by many patients, the greatest limitation appeared to centre about the acquisition of purposeful hand movements' (Wolf et al, 1979). More encouraging results have emerged from an investigation undertaken by Basmajian et al (1982), in relation to 37 patients ranging from 2 to 5 months post-stroke (as opposed to a stroke duration of more than 6 months in patients in the foregoing studies). In this study the greatest functional recovery was observed in patients with severe symptoms treated during the early recovery phase (2 to 3 months post-stroke) and in those having mild symptoms of 4 to 5 months stroke duration.

It has been estimated that only 5% of patients regain meaningful function of the upper limb following stroke illness (Gowland, 1982). The non-functioning arm of the remaining 95% of patients presents one of the greatest challenges in stroke rehabilitation. The studies presented here demonstrate the effectiveness of biofeedback in the re-training of proximal limb musculature, and the value of shoulder and elbow control even in the absence of hand function should not be underestimated. Patients appreciate the fact that the arm presents a more normal appearance, especially in cases where spasticity was previously an overriding factor; they find they can dress more easily and the ability to alter arm position often means a reduction in discomfort. The problem of poor hand function constitutes an area in which intensive research is required. The results of biofeedback therapy at 2 to 3 months post-stroke may be perceived as indicating a need for research into its application in the immediate post-CVA stage (Basmajian et al, 1982). Controlled studies of this nature are yet to be reported.

The lower limb

Biofeedback research in relation to the lower limb in hemiplegic patients has been focused primarily upon the re-activation of paretic anterior tibial muscles and the release of spasticity of the calf muscles. One of the first studies related to the former was undertaken by Johnston and Garton (1973). Patients were trained initially in a rehabilitation setting and when they had grasped the technique they were given small portable units to continue self-treatment at home. The authors reported functional improvement in 7 of the 10 patients treated, 3 of whom were able to discard a previously worn short leg brace.

This form of design in which the patient acted as his own control was used in several succeeding studies. The first controlled study to evaluate the effects of biofeedback therapy was carried out by Basmajian and associates. It also was designed to re-educate the anterior tibial muscles. In their study, the majority of patients had sustained a cerebrovascular lesion at least six months previously. All were treated three times per week for a period of five weeks. Patients in the experimental group received therapeutic exercise plus biofeedback, while patients in the control group received a similar time allocation for therapeutic exercise only. Parameters assessed before and after treatment included range of active movement in the ankle joint and strength of the dorsiflexor muscles. Results at the end of the trial showed that the increase in the range of motion and in muscle strength was approximately twice as great in the biofeedback group (Basmajian et al, 1975). These findings were later challenged since certain dissimilarities existed between the groups in relation to the duration of the stroke and in the interval between initial and final assessments (Fish et al, 1976), but comparable studies elsewhere have demonstrated similar outcomes. These include investigations undertaken by Wolf et al (1979) and by Burnside et al (1982). Interesting results emerged in follow-up assessments in both of these trials. Burnside and fellow workers found significantly greater improvement in muscle strength in the experimental group, but similar improvements by both groups in range of motion of the ankle joint and in gait when assessed at the end of the trial. Six weeks later, however, these improvements had been maintained by the biofeedback group only. In Wolf's study, follow-up assessments for patients treated by biofeedback were carried out over a period of 12 months for 26 patients. The grades achieved at the end of the treatment programme were maintained by all except one patient who had sustained further transient ischaemic attacks (Wolf et al, 1980). This retention of learning indicates an important aspect in rehabilitation, and in relation to biofeedback is one which merits further investigation.

Overriding spasticity in the lower limb constitutes one of the greatest hindrances to the restoration of normal gait, and its reduction has been the subject of several studies using biofeedback. A single case study presented by Amato et al (1973) is one of the earliest in this series. A young man having marked spasticity in the gastrocnemius muscle was treated for a period of two months. As the spasticity was gradually controlled, the patient acquired a corresponding increase in dorsiflexion of the ankle joint, with improvement in function of the anterior tibial muscles. This resulted in a more functional gait pattern, the patient being able to place the foot flat on the ground from heel strike to mid stance. A more specific study designed to train inhibitory control of spasticity in the peroneus longus muscle has been recorded by Swann et al (1974). Seven subjects who exhibited undesired activity in this muscle on extension of the knee were selected for treatment which involved both EMG biofeedback and exercise. Subjects received a 10 minutes session with each form of treatment with a 5 minute rest period in between, the order of treatments being reversed daily. At the end of two weeks, results indicated more effective inhibitory control under biofeedback conditions, but since it is highly probable that there would be some carry-over from one form of treatment to the other the validity of these results has been questioned (Keefe & Surwit, 1978).

The dual problem of paresis and spasticity in agonist and antagonist muscles of the lower limb is well known. Biofeedback has been applied in this situation in order to inhibit spasticity prior to, or simultaneously with the re-activation of the paretic muscles (Wolf et al, 1979; Burnside et al, 1982). In Wolf's study, success in training control of spasticity was gained by applying biofeedback techniques in a progressive sequence from distal to more proximal musculature. Present day neurophysiological approaches to the treatment of the hemiplegic patient emphasise the value of inhibition of spasticity at 'key points of control' in order to reduce muscle hypertonus throughout the entire limb (Bobath, 1978). To date, little or no evidence has been produced to suggest a similar effect using biofeedback, yet this would appear to be a prime factor in neurological rehabilitation and a most relevant aspect of biofeedback research.

Trunk

The importance of trunk control in normal movement cannot be overemphasised, yet investigations to determine the role of biofeedback in the re-education of the trunk have been extremely few. In a pioneer study carried out by Woolley-Hart and associates, the lateral trunk muscles of the affected side were monitored by electrodes positioned just above the iliac crest. Subjects were trained to relax these muscles and allow the pelvis to drop during the swing phase of gait in order to counteract the typical 'hip-hitching' pattern of the hemiplegic patient. During the stance phase, an increase in activity indicated the transference of weight over the affected leg. Results in this study were encouraging; four of the five patients acquired a more normal gait pattern as a result of treatment (Woolley-Hart et al, 1978).

Oro-facial function

Biofeedback has proved to be an effective adjunct to more established techniques in the re-training of the muscles of facial expression following facial nerve palsy (Booker et al, 1969; Brown et al, 1978), and in upper motor neurone lesions (Huffman, 1978). In the latter study, three hemiplegic and one quadriplegic patient received daily training sessions with the use of visual feedback from a mirror for one week. Two patients then changed to biofeedback training while the remaining two continued with conventional mirror feedback. Results at the end of two weeks, evaluated in terms of the ability to develop voluntary symmetrical control of the orbicularis oris muscle during specified movements, indicated gains three times as great for the biofeedback group.

With few exceptions, research programmes designed to investigate the uses of EMG biofeedback in hemiplegic rehabilitation have demonstrated a positive value for this adjunct to therapy. The records noted here indicate the major areas which have been explored, but many of these investigations may be regarded as little more than pilot studies. Without exception, each author stresses the need for further research, and indications of factors which merit investigation are frequently stated.

PRINCIPLES OF BIOFEEDBACK RESEARCH

Certain fundamental principles are essential in any research investigation and a consideration of these in relation to studies which have been published is advisable for the physiotherapist planning to set up a research project.

Research design

As the numbers of biofeedback trials have increased, so more sophisticated research designs have emerged. Patients whose rehabilitation progress had stabilised served as their own controls in early studies (Marinacci & Horande, 1960; Andrews, 1964; Johnston & Garton, 1973). Functional improvement was attained, but it is impossible in this type of design to differentiate between the contribution of biofeedback and the contribution of the many other variables to treatment outcome. Controlled studies involving two or more groups of patients have more recently been undertaken (Basmajian et al, 1976; Burnside et al, 1982). Ideally the two groups should have matched patient samples, in as far as this is possible in neurological rehabilitation, and should receive identical treatment apart from the presence or absence of feedback. A modified cross-over design was used by Huffman (1978). Two groups of patients received similar therapy for one week. Then while one group continued with exercise therapy for a further week, the second group had the added benefit of biofeedback therapy. A third tier to this programme was added in research undertaken by Santee et al (1980), in which patients received first exercise therapy, then exercise therapy plus biofeedback, and finally a monetary incentive was added to the biofeedback training. Maximum gains were achieved under the third form of treatment!

Results obtained from controlled studies involving a large number of patients carry greater validity than those from uncontrolled trials. This fact should not however deter the physiotherapist in a small rehabilitation unit from incorporating biofeedback into her treatment programme if it is considered to be beneficial for selected patients. Important variables (as noted under Patient characteristics) should be kept in mind, and patients undergoing biofeedback and non-biofeedback treatment should be matched when possible. The cumulative evidence from such small-scale studies cannot be ignored.

Patient characteristics

Much research has been carried out in order to determine patient characteristics which may help to predict the outcome of biofeedback therapy. One of the most comprehensive studies in this area undertaken by Wolf and co-workers, demonstrated no significant correlation between age, sex, side affected and outcome (Wolf et al, 1979). These findings are supported by several other writers (Brudny et al, 1976; Shiavi et al, 1979; Smith, 1979). Unanimous agreement has not been obtained in relation to other characteristics, the chief of which are as follows:

Duration of stroke

Certain trends between the duration of stroke and outcome have been observed, but no statistically significant correlations have emerged. Long duration illness and extended rehabilitation programmes were found to mitigate against a good recovery in the upper limb (Wolf et al, 1979; Skelly, 1980; Hurd, 1980). In contrast, caution regarding the application of biofeedback therapy during the early post-stroke phase has been urged by Baker (1979), who reported that such patients appear to progress slowly and experience difficulty in re-learning muscular control. One suggested explanation for this paradox is that the recently injured brain is unable to cope with the concentration and conscious thought demanded by biofeedback treatment. Findings reported by Basmajian et al (1982, see p. 133) regarding patients treated two or three months following a stroke would, however, encourage continued research during these early recovery stages. Successful outcomes in lower limb re-education have been achieved in patients at all stages of post-stroke rehabilitation, and there would appear to be no significant difference in degree of recovery between early treatment and late treatment groups (Wolf et al, 1979; Burnside et al, 1982).

Sensory status

Sensory deficit in hemiplegia has long been recognised as a barrier to recovery (Twitchell, 1957), and for patients in this category EMG biofeedback would appear to have special value. While fine manipulative skills cannot be restored in the absence of tactile and proprioceptive awareness, successful re-education of voluntary movement of the more proximal joints of the upper limb has been achieved. A controlled study undertaken by Skelly and Kenedi (1982) to evaluate EMG biofeedback in the restoration of shoulder control in patients without sensation, demonstrated improvement in both groups of patients with no significant difference in response between the two groups. Similar findings were obtained by Smith (1979), but Wolf et al (1979) reported a high proportion of failure outcomes in patients with sensory loss. These apparently contradictory results may be due to differences in assessment procedures, which in the latter study demanded normal hand function for success grades to be allocated.

The lower limb is less dependent on feedback for function than the upper limb. This is illustrated in a single case study reported by Skelly (1983). The patient, a 60-year-old woman, had good recovery of motor power following stroke, but complete loss of sensation of the lower part of the leg resulted in an unstable, inverted foot. Following four weeks of therapy, the patient was able to walk on level surfaces with a normal plantigrade foot. On re-assessment two years later this ability was retained. The patient was able to walk at a near normal pace, and used a walking stick only when negotiating uneven ground in her garden. She lived an active life and was able to return to voluntary work in a nearby hospital. Sensory and proprioceptive loss in her leg remained unaltered.

Functional levels

Patients whose symptoms are mild or who have already attained a moderate level of ability appear to gain the greatest benefit from EMG biofeedback. A highly significant correlation ($p > 0.01$) between initial and final assessment grades was reported by Skelly and Kenedi (1982). A similar finding emerged from a study by Basmajian and associates which led to the recommendation, 'while humanitarian considerations suggest that all patients should have biofeedback, this is unrealistic in research. Hence further studies should be based upon the effect of new therapy on patients who have the greatest likelihood of measureable recovery.' (Basmajian et al, 1982).

Measurement

Measurement of outcome in biofeedback research poses one of its most difficult problems, a problem which is accentuated when the many variables associated with stroke rehabilitation are superimposed. Rigidly controlled studies may help to eliminate variables such as the patient-therapist interaction and the stimulus of new electronic gadgetry. Careful selection of patients who have a good standard of general fitness and who are more than six months post-stroke will minimise the improvement due to spontaneous recovery but will never rule it out completely. The presence or absence of spasticity is likely to affect outcome, as are other factors such as motivation and perception. Parameters selected for assessment purposes have included muscle strength, range of active motion, and integrated EMG activity. Positive achievement in each of these areas is to be commended, but while they may accurately reflect the value of biofeedback as a treatment modality for that chosen parameter, they have not always resulted in functional improvement. The latter must always remain a priority in hemiplegic research. Lower limb function has been widely assessed in relation to gait, and improvement has been achieved by many patients. This has been particularly evident in those who have been able to discard a lower limb orthosis. Assessment of gait by visual observation alone is inevitably subjective, especially if carried out by the therapist performing the treatment. Independent assessors should be used if possible to eliminate any bias in the evaluation process and so give greater validity to the results. Biofeedback trials based upon more objective measurements such as cadence, weightbearing, speed of walking and distance covered should yield interesting information, but such studies are still to be reported.

In the assessment of upper limb function, care should be taken to differentiate between function of the limb as a whole, and manual function and dexterity. Assessment scales which rely heavily upon the latter give no credit for increases in the control of the more proximal joints. Tests which are based upon an ascending scale of abilities related to the function of the entire arm and which follow the normal sequence of restoration of upper limb function in the stroke patient are to be preferred. The upper extremity function test (UEFT) devised by Carroll has been designed on this basis (Carroll, 1965). The experienced physiotherapist should be encouraged to devise her own assessment scales, based upon her individual expertise and knowledge.

Retention of learning is essential if goals realised at the end of the treatment programme are to be maintained. Follow-up assessments over a period of one or two years are desirable if this aspect of biofeedback training is to be evaluated.

Recording

Meticulous record keeping is essential if research is to be valid. Recording may take a variety of forms, but the written record is still the most commonly used. Factual information regarding the individual characteristics of the patient must be noted. The use of charts and/or numerical rating systems in the assessment of function will help to direct the attention of the evaluator to specific aspects and should help to minimise subjective variations. Films and video recordings are widely used, but it should be realised that these do not lend themselves to objective analysis unless taken in conjunction with devices designed to record distance, space and timing. More sophisticated electronic apparatus, such as Polgon for recording joint angles and force plates to measure weight transference and stance, are becoming more widely available and yield accurate results.

Appropriate collection and analysis of data is imperative if significant improvements are to be demonstrated. Unless the researcher is competent in this area, advice should be obtained from a statistician prior to the commencement of the research programme, to ensure that measurements recorded are relevant to the investigation and will yield satisfactory data for analytical purposes.

BIOFEEDBACK—MODE OF ACTION

The efficacy of EMG biofeedback in the training of muscular control has perhaps been most clearly demonstrated in the training of single motor units. This fine control of voluntary movement has been achieved by many subjects who, following a few short sessions using biofeedback, have been able to activate isolated motor units on command (Basmajian, 1979). The mechanism by which this has been accomplished is unclear but the fact is indisputable. The efficacy of EMG biofeedback in the re-training of movement in the hemiplegic patient has also been well documented, yet relatively few attempts have been made to formulate hypotheses upon which its mode of action may be based.

Success in the re-training of movement in the hemiplegic patient has normally been attributed to the opening up of pathways in the central nervous system which have survived damage and have lain dormant. On this assumption researchers have concluded that biofeedback is an effective tool to aid patients to discover and use these pathways (Basmajian, 1981). Others have equated biofeedback training with operant conditioning, (Shapiro & Schwartz, 1972; Huffman, 1978). This theory has been refuted by Wolf (1979) who noted the dissimilarities between these two techniques. Serious consideration of the mode of action of EMG biofeedback must be undertaken in conjunction with present day concepts regarding the acquisition and control of skilled movements. This topic has undergone extensive research in recent years, but only a brief outline of the major hypotheses can be considered in this chapter.

Sensory engram theory

This theory is based upon the centrality of sensory feedback in the control of voluntary movement. During the performance of purposeful movement, information from the sensory receptors is relayed to the CNS, thus providing an immediate awareness of both the on-going activity within the body and also of the outcome of that activity. A memory store of the correct pattern of afferent impulses associated with that movement is laid down. This pattern or engram can serve as a frame of reference for subsequent movements. Its mode of action in the initiation and control of voluntary movement has been summarised as follows, 'sensory information arising from a particular movement serves to instigate the next movement in the series . . . during the acquisition and performance of a skill, the sensory feedback is used in a comparator system not only in the control of the on-going response but also in providing the system with a basis for the correction and modification of the response' (Glencross, 1978). Sensory engrams are thus seen as the major factor in a closed-loop system, having the capacity to initiate, evaluate and modify performance.

This theory is used as a basis for Wolf's model explaining the mode of action of EMG biofeedback (Wolf, 1979). Wolf supports the concept that activation of the sensory engram will initiate a chain of events leading to activation of the motor system, the cerebellum acting as the comparator to sample and modify performance as required. In his model, the muscle spindle is regarded as the main proprioceptive organ. Imbalance in motor control of the alpha and gamma motor neurones arising from lesions within the CNS will result in hypo- or hyper-sensitivity of the muscle spindle. Sensory information arising from these organs will therefore be inaccurate, making the detection of errors by the cerebellum an impossibility.

The visual and auditory systems of the body are noted to have synaptic links with the cerebellum, and Wolf sees these as the obvious temporary pathways to be used as a replacement for the normal proprioceptive information channels. The required modifications to motor output may then be instigated. He further suggests that the ability of patients to discard electronic feedback following training, is indicative of the establishment of an increasingly reliable linkage between the sensory engram and functionally transmitting cells, thus allowing patients to rely once more upon proprioceptive feedback. Wolf's hypothesis may be summed up in his assertion that the key to re-acquiring motor control in neuro-logical patients rests in re-establishing proper proprioceptive behaviour.

The value of correct sensory input in stroke rehabilitation is widely recognised. Brodal (1973) speaks from his own experience as he relates how passive movement helped to facilitate subsequent active contraction of the relevant muscles. The need for reducing spasticity in antagonistic muscles prior to active or assisted active movement in order to give the patient the correct 'feel' of move-ment is also well documented (Bobath, 1978). Wolf's model supports these concepts, and provides an acceptable hypothesis to account for successful re-training of movement in subjects whose proprioceptive pathways are intact. It offers no explanation, however, for the recovery of movement in patients who have experi-enced complete loss of sensation, but who have acquired a func-tional degree of control in selected movements. For them, an alternative explanation must be sought.

Movement without sensation

The acquisition of functional movement in the absence of proprio-ceptive feedback has been clearly demonstrated in experimental situations. In a series of animal studies where proprioceptive input was ablated by posterior rhizotomy, Taub and Berman (1965) have reported on the ability of monkeys to learn to execute gross, purposeful movements. Related research has shown enhancement of movement following bi-lateral de-afferentation (Knapp et al, 1963). These results suggest a control system which relies upon motor output rather than upon sensory input.

Motor engram theories

The motor engram or outflow hypothesis maintains that skilled movements are organised and initiated by a central control process, and knowledge of the movement results from the monitoring of the efferent or output signal, rather than upon any peripheral sensory input (Glencross, 1979). Researchers supporting this hypothesis have argued that certain motor sequences, such as the finger move-ments in typing or in playing a piano, occur too rapidly to allow for control mediated by sensory feedback loops and their associated chain reactions (Lashley, 1951). A similar argument applies to fast ball games in which ballistic movements to kick or catch a ball occur in such a rapid sequence that no time is allowed for modification via sensory loops.

Brodal (1973) in 'Self-Observations after a Stroke' relates his difficulty in tying a bow tie, which required 7–10 attempts before success was achieved. He writes, 'The appropriate finger movements were difficult to perform with sufficient strength, speed and coordination, but it was quite obvious to the patient that the main reason for the failure was something else. Under normal conditions the necessary numerous small delicate movements had followed each other in the proper sequence almost automatically, and the act of tying when first started had proceeded without much conscious attention. Subjectively the patient felt as if he had to stop because 'his fingers did not know the next move'. He had the same feeling as when one recites a poem or sings a song and gets lost. The only way is to start from the beginning. It was felt as if the delay in the succession of movements (due to paresis and spasticity) interrupted a chain of more or less automatic movements. Consciously directing attention to the finger movements did not improve the performance; on the contrary it made it quite impossible.'

The motor engram theory has been adopted by Laszlo and Bairstow (1971) in support of their servo-systems model in which all data relevant to a particular task is stored in a perceptual/processing centre referred to as the 'Standard'. The Standard controls a subsidiary Motor Programme Unit which selects the appropriate motor response and a movement is effected. The standard receives information from the peripheral sensory feedback loop which detects errors in the response. It also receives information from the 'efference copy' or central feedback loop which acts within the central nervous system and monitors the command signal, i.e. the sequence of efferent motor impulses, with complete disregard for the consequences of the movement. The authors contend that the efference copy loop is in itself sufficient to maintain performance after learning has occurred in relatively simple tasks. With efference copy, increase and decrease in the rate of performance may be gained, but there can be no error detection or correction in the absence of peripheral feedback, therefore no improvement in the quality of performance. This theory would appear to offer a workable hypothesis upon which the mode of action of EMG biofeedback training in patients with sensory loss may be based. The visual and auditory signals provide the required peripheral feedback to the Standard which in turn directs the Motor Programme outflow, (Fig. 6.2). Discrepancies between the desired and the actual

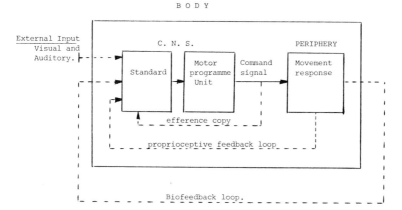

Fig. 6.2 Diagrammatic representation of efference copy, proprioceptive and biofeedback loops carrying information to the Standard.

outcome may be recognised and corrected. With repetition, predictable sequences of movement are gradually formed into motor impulse sub-routines with a shift in control from the Standard to the Motor Programme level.

Pew (1966) has demonstrated that feedback dependence during the early stages of skill acquisition is gradually phased out as motor execution becomes more confident and precise. In using EMG biofeedback, it is suggested that when the correct sequences of motor outflow have been learned, efference copy feedback is adequate to ensure its continuance, and electronic feedback may be withdrawn. In simple repetitive movements such as dorsiflexion of the foot in the gait cycle, such learning can lead to adequate control for normal walking on flat surfaces without the application of any external orthotic device. Efference copy and visual feedback may be used jointly in directing movements of the upper limb. It is recognised that precision and fine co-ordination will be lacking in movements re-trained in the absence of sensation. Feedback-dependent activities, such as doing up small buttons or controlling the accelerator of a car, will be either clumsy or even impossible.

While both sensory and motor engram hypotheses offer control models which may to some extent explain the mode of action of EMG biofeedback, it would be unrealistic to accept them as the final authority on this form of re-training. Too many gaps in knowledge remain. These theories in themselves do not explain the many complexities inherent in highly skilled movements. Many recent hypotheses favour hierarchial systems of control, in which centres at varying levels within the central nervous system interact with each other both in the learning of novel skills and in the control of semi-automatic activities of everyday life (MacKay, 1982; Glencross, 1976). These tend to be based upon scientific experiment and observation rather than upon known neuroanatomical and neurophysiological connections within the central nervous system. They offer interesting areas for study and for speculation for the clinician seeking to find an answer to the many problems associated with the re-learning of movement in the hemiplegic patient.

APPENDIX: EMG BIOFEEDBACK—EQUIPMENT AND PRINCIPLES OF APPLICATION

The EMG signal

When a muscle contracts, a series of electrochemical changes occur at the neuromuscular junction and in the myofibrils. In electromyography, the related minute potentials are detected and amplified. The resulting signal may be processed in a variety of ways. It may be displayed on an oscilloscope as a series of spike potentials. It may be rectified and integrated to give a meter reading or a digital count. It may be processed to produce an auditory tone or to operate a sequential series of light bulbs. The EMG signal is not directly proportional to the degree of muscle tension. It will vary according to the type of contraction, i.e. isometric or isotonic, and also with the speed of contraction. For re-education purposes, however, the integrated EMG signal may be assumed to be an appropriate indication of the functional activity of muscle. In EMG biofeedback the signal is displayed to the patient, so that with training he may learn to increase or decrease the electrical activity and so gain control over the level of tone in the muscles being monitored.

BIOFEEDBACK EQUIPMENT

The extensive range of biofeedback equipment currently available can appear confusing, making selection difficult. The choice of a model may be limited by financial constraints, but careful consideration of the field of operation is advisable prior to purchase. For serious research, the larger models are the units of choice. They normally afford greater accuracy of signal processing and a wider variety of feedback devices including series of light bulbs and/or digital displays. Many models are manufactured for use in conjunction with optional equipment such as oscilloscope displays and computers for on-line recording and analysis of data. This type of apparatus is usually designed for use in a fixed location.

Medium-sized units weighing just a few pounds are popular, and have proved very satisfactory for research and for rehabilitation purposes. Models of this type (Fig. 6.3) normally offer feedback in both auditory and visual modes. They are easily portable and when supplied with a carrying case can be used for gait re-training in addition to use in more fixed situations. Pocket-sized units are designed for the ambulant patient and frequently offer auditory feedback only. Their simplicity of operation makes them especially suitable for self-treatment by patients following discharge from hospital. Whatever model is selected, the following features are essential for re-education purposes.

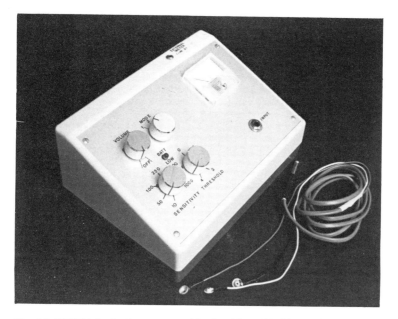

Fig. 6.3 EMG biofeedback apparatus with silver/silver chloride cup electrodes.

Feedback

Meters displaying the integrated EMG signal will be found on all but the smallest models, and are essential not only for the patient but also to give the therapist a precise indication of the levels of muscular activity. The meter should be controlled by a sensitivity device, and ideally should encompass a range from 0 to 1000 microvolts. Surface recordings of EMG levels in everyday activities rarely exceed 600 microvolts but higher voltages may be obtained. At the other extreme, the fully relaxed muscle is electrically silent, so sensitivity at lower levels of output is essential. Alternate forms of visual display include series of light bulbs or lights of varying colours which are operated sequentially with increasing levels of EMG activity.

Auditory feedback will usually give a choice of two or more sound effects. It may take the form of a buzzing tone which increases in pitch, or alternatively a short sharp click may be obtainable, the rate of clicks varying according to the intensity of the signal. The effectiveness of both visual and audio feedback will depend on patient interests and characteristics. Defects of vision and hearing are common in the population under consideration and frequently influence the preferred form of feedback.

Threshold level control

A variable threshold device allows the setting of a specific level of activity which must be exceeded before the audio or visual feedback is activated. When used in reverse, it determines the level for the reduction in muscle tone before electrical silence is achieved. In this way, the patient's responses may be 'shaped' to encourage subtle increases or decreases in muscular contraction.

Electrodes

Early EMG feedback treatment was carried out using concentric needle electrodes but these were soon discontinued in favour of surface electrodes. Two types of surface electrode are commonly available. Silver/silver chloride cup electrodes, as seen in Figure 6.3 are obtainable in varying sizes The smaller sizes are valuable in the monitoring of small muscles such as the intrinsic hand muscles. These electrodes may be used repeatedly and will give long service if properly handled and cleaned after use. Disposable electrodes are manufactured from inexpensive materials and normally consist of a metal disc 10 mm to 12 mm in diameter, embedded in an adhesive plastic ring. They are convenient to use but the fine wire connections are easily damaged. Surface electrodes are ideal when monitoring large superficial muscles such as the deltoid, but in the re-education of deeply placed muscles such as the peroneus longus, it is difficult to eliminate pick-up from adjacent muscles. In such situations very specific placement of electrodes will be essential, but with care, satisfactory feedback is usually obtainable.

Leads

Leads should be long enough to permit freedom of movement but if too long, the greater capacitance will tend to reduce the accuracy of the signal. Leads measuring from 1 to $1\frac{1}{2}$ meters in length are optimal for most purposes. Movement of the leads during dynamic training is inevitable, but this should be kept to a minimum to reduce artefact in the signal. The use of pre-amplification at the electrode site will also reduce distortion of the signal. This facility is not normally available with portable apparatus but it is highly recommended for research involving accurate measurement of the integrated EMG signal.

PRINCIPLES OF APPLICATION

Accurate assessment of the patient is essential in order to determine priorities in treatment, to obtain baseline data for evaluation purposes, and to set realistic goals. The concept of biofeedback must be explained to the patient and the apparatus demonstrated. The principles of working are usually grasped even by patients suffering from receptive aphasia, following a demonstration of feedback either by the physiotherapist or by attaching the electrodes to the patient's sound limb for practice purposes. As a rule only one muscle is selected for feedback, although simultaneous monitoring of two muscle groups using audio feedback for one group and visual for the other has been satisfactorily performed (Prevo et al, 1982) Factors such as the superficiality of muscle fibres and the impingement of adjacent muscles must be considered when determining the electrode site. Guidelines for the placement of electrodes in specific muscle re-training have been documented (Wolf, 1978; Kelly et al, 1979) but some element of trial and error is inevitable in determining the optimum site for individual patients.

Skin preparation

Electrical impedance at the electrode/skin interface must be reduced to a minimum. The skin is thoroughly cleaned with spirit then rubbed briskly or abraded lightly with fine sandpaper to remove dead cells. Hairs are removed by shaving. Conducting gel is then applied to the two active electrodes which are taped firmly into position. A ground electrode is likewise attached at a point slightly removed from the active electrodes. Certain authorities recommend a position over a non-muscular area such as the sternum or the medial surface of the tibia, but this is not always possible nor is it essential. In ambulatory situations leads may be taped to the patient's skin or attached to clothing to prevent unnecessary artefact.

Biofeedback techniques

In the re-training of paretic muscles, electrodes are initially widely spaced to allow for maximum pick-up, and a low threshold level set to permit easy activation of the feedback device. Once this is achieved, the threshold level is progressively raised and the spacing reduced so that greater recruitment of motor units is required to produce the same feedback response. Threshold levels must set a target within the patient's capabilities otherwise excessive effort may lead to the production of undesirable total synergy patterns of movement. The patient's efforts are therefore shaped to produce increasing levels of muscular contraction. In the reduction of spasticity, similar techniques are employed but in a reversed order of application.

Feedback is normally offered in both auditory and visual modes. Auditory feedback allows the patient freedom of vision to observe the movement directly or to relate to the environment, essential in the re-training of gait. Patients whose previous experience allows them to appreciate the significance of microvolt levels on a meter find greater stimulation from this modality. Verbal reinforcement for a correct response may be used to heighten the patient's awareness and to augment feedback. Biofeedback techniques which have proved valuable in the re-training of specific functions have been well documented (de Bacher, 1979; Baker & Wolf, 1979), but each therapist will need to experiment and utilise her own individual expertise.

Physiotherapy techniques

Biofeedback is no substitute for dynamic physiotherapy, but it should be fully integrated into the normal physiotherapy programme. The complete range and variety of therapeutic skills should still be applied. A stereotyped approach using inflexible positioning or a set sequence of rehabilitation measures may help to eliminate variables in the research programme but may not be in the best interests of the patient. Modifications in tactile stimulation may be necessary due to the placement of electrodes, and lead lengths may restrict gross movement patterns. The use of variations in positioning, reflex stimulation, inhibition, bi-lateral movements, weight-bearing stimuli, pressure tapping and other such techniques should be applied as appropriate. Biofeedback re-education should not be regarded merely as a method of training a specific muscle. Rather, target muscles should be trained where possible to fulfill their normal role in composite movements and in selective movement patterns. The re-education of the muscles of the lower limb, for example the tibialis anterior, may be undertaken initially in a sitting posture to allow the patient to observe the movement, but after a few attempts he should be encouraged to integrate the action of dorsiflexion into the normal gait cycle (Fig. 6.4). A knowledge of the phasic activity of the muscles of the lower limb in walking is essential if accurate training is to be undertaken. This activity has been well documented (Milner et al, 1971).

Training without feedback should be undertaken at an early stage so that the patient does not become feedback dependent. The visual or auditory signal may be switched off at intervals during treatment sessions while the patient uses mental recall while trying to produce the desired movement. Alternatively, practice without feedback is frequently undertaken at the beginning and the end of treatment sessions.

Biofeedback demands a high level of concentration from both the patient and the therapist, so initially treatment is best carried out in a quiet atmosphere isolated from other distractions. Later, however, it may be desirable to continue training in a more stressful environment to ensure transfer of newly acquired abilities into everyday situations. This is particularly important in the reduction of spasticity, to ensure that low levels of muscle tonus are maintained when walking or performing other activities.

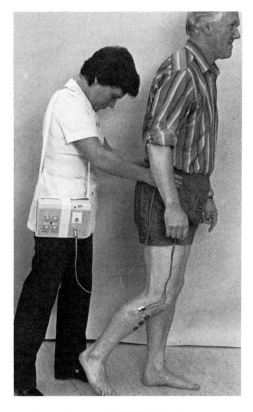

Fig. 6.4 Gait re-training using portable EMG biofeedback apparatus.

Treatment schedules

The frequency and duration of treatment sessions and the extent of the rehabilitation programme will be determined by individual work situations and by patient responses. Treatment is carried out daily if possible, but in many circumstances sessions scheduled three times per week have proved satisfactory. The high degree of concentration required in biofeedback training may result in early fatigue, so treatment sessions should not extend beyond a total of 30–45 minutes duration.

REFERENCES

Amato A, Hermsmeyer C A, Kleinman K M 1973 Use of electromyographic feedback to increase inhibitory control of spastic muscles. Physical Therapy 53: 10, 1063–1066

Andrews J M 1964 Neuromuscular re-education of the hemiplegic with the aid of the electromyograph. Physical Therapy 45: 530–532

Baker M P 1979 Biofeedback in specific muscle re-training. In: Basmajian J V (ed) Biofeedback—principles and practice for clinicians. The Williams and Wilkins Company, Baltimore, ch 7, p 81

Baker M P, Wolf S L 1979 Biofeedback strategies in the physical therapy clinic. In: Basmajian J V (ed) Biofeedback—principles and practice for clinicians. Williams and Wilkins Company, Baltimore, ch 3, p 31

Basmajian J V 1979 Muscles alive, 4th edn. The Williams and Wilkins Company, Baltimore, ch 5, p 115

Basmajian J V 1981 Biofeedback in rehabilitation—a review of principles and practice. Archives of Physical Medicine and Rehabilitation 62: 469–475

Basmajian J V, Kukulka C G, Narayan M G, Takebe K 1975 'Biofeedback treatment of foot-drop after stroke compared with standard rehabilitation technique: Effects on voluntary control and strength'. Archives of Physical Medicine and Rehabilitation 56: 231–236

Basmajian J V, Regenos E M, Baker M P 1977 Rehabilitating stroke patients with biofeedback. Geriatrics 32: 85–88

Basmajian J V, Gowland C, Brandstater M E, Swanson L, Trotter J 1982 E M G feedback treatment of upper limb in hemiplegic stroke patients: a pilot study. Archives of Physical Medicine and Rehabilitation 63: 613–616

Bobath B 1978 Adult hemiplegia—evaluation and treatment, 2nd ed. Heinmann, London

Booker H E, Rubow R T, Coleman P J 1969 Simplified feedback in neuromuscular re-training: an automated approach using electromyographic signals. Archives of Physical Medicine and Rehabilitation 50: 621–625

Brodal A 1973 Self-observation and neuro-anatomical considerations after a stroke. Brain 96: 657–694

Brown D M, Nahai F, Wolf S, Basmajian J V 1978 Electromyographic feedback in the re-education of facial palsy. American Journal of Physical Medicine 57: 183–190

Brudny J, Korein J, Grynbaum B B, Friedmann L W, Weinstein S, Sach-Frankel G, Belandres P V 1976 E M G feedback therapy: review of 114 patients. Archives of Physical Medicine and Rehabilitation 57: 55–61

Burnside I G, Tobias H S, Bursill D 1982 Electromyographic feedback in the remobilisation of stroke patients: a controlled trial. Archives of Physical Medicine and Rehabilitation 63: 217–222

Carroll D 1965 A quantitative test of upper extremity function. Journal of Chronic Diseases 18: 479–491

de Bacher G 1979 Biofeedback in spasticity control. In: Basmajian J V (ed) Biofeedback—principles and practice for clinicians. The Williams and Wilkins Company, Baltimore, ch 6, p 61

Fish D, Mayer N, Herman R 1976 Biofeedback: letters to the editor. Archives of Physical Medicine and Rehabilitation 57:152

Glencross D J 1978 Control and capacity in the study of skill. In: Glencross D J (ed) Phychology and Sport. McGraw-Hill Book Company, Sydney, ch 4, p 172

Gowland C 1982 Recovery of motor function following stroke: profile and predictors. Physiotherapy 34: 77–84

Huffman A L 1978 Biofeedback treatment of orofacial dysfunction: a preliminary study. The American Journal of Occupational Therapy 32: 3, 149–154

Hurd W W, Pegram V, Nepomuceno C 1980 Comparison of actual and simulated

E M G biofeedback in the treatment of the hemiplegic patient. American Journal of Physical Medicine 59: 2, 73–82

Johnston H E, Garton W H 1973 'Muscle re-education in hemiplegia by use of electromyographic device'. Archives of Physical Medicine and Rehabilitation 53: 320–325

Keefe F J, Surwit R S 1978 Electromyographic biofeedback: behavioural treatment of neuromuscular disorders. Journal of Behavioural Medicine 1: 1, 13–24

Kelly J L, Baker M P, Wolf S L 1979 Procedures for E M G biofeedback training in involved upper extremities of hemiplegia patients. Physical Therapy 59:12, 1500–1507

Kleinman K M, Keister M E, Riggin C S, Goldman H, Korol B 1976 Use of EMG feedback to inhibit flexor spasticity and increase active extension in Stroke Patients. Proceedings of the Biofeedback Society of America. 38

Knapp H D, Taub E, Berman A J 1963 Movements in monkeys with deafferented forelimbs. Experimental Neurology 7: 305–315

Kotses H, Glaus K, Bricel S 1977 Muscle relaxation effects on peak expiratory flow rate in asthmatic children. Proceedings of the Biofeedback Research Society, Orlando, Fla

Kristt D A, Engel B T 1975 Learned control of blood pressure in patients with high blood pressure, Circulation 51: 370–378

Lashley K S 1951 The problem of serial order in behaviour. In: Jeffress L A (ed) Cerebral mechanism in behaviour. Wiley, New York

Laszlo J I, Bairstow P J 1979 Accuracy of movement, peripheral feedback and efference copy. Journal of Motor Behaviour 3: 241–252

Lee K–H, Hill E, Johnston R, Smiehorowski T 1976 Myofeedback for muscle re-training in hemiplegic patients. Archives of Physical Medicine and Rehabilitation 57: 588–591

MacKay D G 1982 The problems of flexibility, fluency and speed-accuracy trade-off in skilled behaviour. Psychological Review 89:5, 483–506

Marinacci A A, Horande M 1960 Electromyogram in neuromuscular re-education. Bulletin of the Los Angeles Neurological Society 25:2, 57–71

Middaugh S J, Miller M C 1980 Electromyographic feedback: effect on voluntary contraction in paretic subjects. Archives of Physical Medicine and Rehabilitation 61: 24–29

Milner M, Basmajian J V, Quanbury A O 1971 Multifactoral analysis of walking by electromyography and computer. American Journal of Physical Medicine 50: 235–258

Nafpliotis H 1976 Electromyographic feedback to improve ankle dorsiflexion, wrist extension and hand grasp. Physical Therapy 56: 821–825

Pew R W 1966 Acquisition of hierarchical control over the temporal organisation of a skill. Journal of Experimental Psychology 71: 764–771

Prevo A J H, Visser S L, Vogelaar T W 1982 Effect of EMG feedback on paretic muscle and abnormal co-contraction in the hemiplegic arm, compared with conventional physical therapy. Scandinavian Journal of Rehabilitation Medicine 14: 121–131

Santee J L, Keister M E, Kleinman K M 1980 Incentives to enhance the effects of electromyographic feedback training in stroke patients. Biofeedback and Self-regulation 5:1, 51–56

Sargent J D, Green E E, Walters E D 1972 The use of autogenic feedback training in a pilot study of migraine and tension headaches. Headache 12: 120–124

Shapiro D, Schwartz G E 1972 Biofeedback and visceral learning: clinical applications. Seminars in Psychiatry 4: 171–184

Shiavi R G, Champion S A, Freeman F R, Bugel H J 1979 Efficacy of myofeedback therapy in regaining control of lower extremity musculature following stroke. American Journal of Physical Medicine 58:4, 185–194

Skelly A M 1980 Applications of EMG biofeedback in rehabilitation. M. Sc. Thesis, University of Strathclyde (unpublished)

Skelly A M 1983 Biofeedback in stroke rehabilitation. Research in rehabilitation/First European Conference, Scientific Programme/Abstracts

Skelly A M, Kenedi R M 1982 EMG feedback therapy in the re-education of the Hemiplegic shoulder in patients with sensory loss, Physiotherapy 68:2, 34–38

Smith K N 1979 Biofeedback in stroke. Australian Journal of Physiotherapy 25:4, 155–161

Swaan D, van Wieringen P C W, Fokkema S D 1974 Auditory electromyographic feedback therapy to inhibit undesired motor activity. Archives of Physical Medicine and Rehabilitation 55:6, 251–254

Taub E, Berman A J 1968 Movement and learning in the absence of sensory feedback. In: Freedman S J (ed) The neuropsychology of spatially oriented behaviour. Dorsey Press, Homewood, Illinois

Twitchell T E 1957 The prognosis of motor recovery in hemiplegia. Bulletin of Tufts—New England Medical Centre 3: 146–149.

Wolf S L 1979 Anatomical and physiological basis for biofeedback. In: Basmajian J V (ed) Biofeedback—principles and practice for clinicians. Williams and Wilkins Company, Baltimore, ch 2, p 5

Wolf S L, Baker M P, Kelly J L 1979 EMG biofeedback in stroke: effect of patient characteristics. Archives of Physical Medicine and Rehabilitation 60: 96–102

Wolf S L, Baker M P, Kelly J L 1980 EMG biofeedback in stroke: a 1-year follow-up on the effect of patient characteristics. Archives of Physical Medicine and Rehabilitation 61: 351–355

Woolley-Hart A, Musa I, Rodger E 1977 The use of electromyographic biofeedback in the re-training of gait following stroke. Chest, Heart and Stroke Journal 77/78: 2–4

The application of motor learning theory

INTRODUCTION

In Canada each year, one in every 500 people develop stroke and it has been estimated that stroke patients occupy 2 million hospital days stay in Canada per annum (Pryse-Phillips & Murray, 1982). Stroke has been cited as the third leading cause of death and the chief cause of long-term disability in the United States (McCann & Culbertson, 1976) as well as one of the major causes of disability in elderly populations.

The medical and surgical treatment of completed stroke is limited and the primary therapeutic approach of the resultant residual deficits has been directed towards the rehabilitation of the survivor (Brocklehurst et al, 1978).

Physiotherapists are generally considered to be fundamental members of the stroke rehabilitation team (Isaacs, 1978; Redford & Harris, 1980; Stonnington, 1980). The role of physiotherapy, in general terms, has the objective of restoring more normal function and is particularly involved in the assessment, treatment and management of disorders of movement (Carr & Shepherd, 1980; Atkinson, 1982). Physiotherapy in the management of stroke consists mainly of procedures of therapeutic exercise, and a variety of models have been proposed by several workers to deal effectively with the rehabilitation of people suffering from neurological dysfunction including stroke (Stockmeyer, 1967; Voss, 1967; Brunnstrom, 1970; Bobath, 1977). These approaches have been analysed by several authors including Gonella et al (1978) who reduced the principles of all techniques to four common denominators while conceding differences in conceptual emphasis and procedure. The four common factors described were: (1) the use of sensory input to facilitate or inhibit CNS activity; (2) the application of neurodevelopmental concepts; (3) the application of skilled manual techniques; and (4) the use of concepts from the psychology of learning. It is the purpose of this chapter to elaborate on the latter factor and apply principles from the field of motor skills acquisition to the physiotherapeutic management of stroke.

In the theoretical framework of physiotherapy approaches, Knott and Voss (1967) have acknowledged that motor learning was part of the basis of the proprioceptive neuromuscular facilitation procedures and Gonnella (1978, 1980) has also discussed the objective of behaviour change in physiotherapy through attention to mechanisms of learning. More recently, several authors such as Turnbull (1982) and Carr and Shephard (1983) have presented the re-education of people with neurological deficit in a learning framework.

HUMAN LEARNING

To maximise the relearning of functional movement it is necessary for physiotherapists to have a clear understanding of learning approaches and processes, particularly in the area of motor skill acquisition.

Learning has been defined by Sage (1977) as 'the internal process assumed to occur whenever a change in performance, not due to maturation or fatigue, exhibits itself.'

Early models of learning subscribed to a behaviouristic orientation. The work of Pavlov, Thorndike, Hull and Skinner emphasised stimulus/response relationships and were largely experimental, emphasising repeatibility, prediction and the manipulation of specific variables. It was shown quite clearly that specific stimulus/response bonds could be strengthened by the attention to such principles as reinforcement, punishment and contiguity. This behaviouristic orientation laid the foundation for the study of learning psychology, but its application to humans was severely limited due to the fact that this approach tended to pay little attention to the processing organism. Additionally, the variables which affect learning in humans cannot be adequately controlled in the same way as that of lower life forms in the laboratory setting.

During the 1960s a new learning orientation began to emerge and has gained widespread subscription. The cognitive orientation of learning has, as the predominant feature, a recognition of the uniqueness of the learner and has been defined as 'any change in one's potential for seeing, thinking, feeling and doing through experiences partly perceptual, partly intellectual, partly emotional and partly motor.'

It is therefore important that human learning is viewed as an entity which is unique to each person, which is not necessarily observable and which is very difficult to predict and control.

DOMAINS OF LEARNING

For purposes of description, learning can be said to occur in three psychological domains (Magill, 1980). The cognitive domain deals with intellectual concepts such as knowledge, understanding and problem solving (Bloom et al, 1956), while the affective domain accounts for such learning as social skills, emotion and moral judgement (Krathwohl et al, 1964). The psychomotor domain encompasses the acquisition of skills which are largely motor but which depend heavily on sensori-perceptual-motor relationships. Activities included under this category range from sophisticated sporting skills through vocational tasks to activities of daily living. It would seem that the psychomotor domain would be the learning area of most relevance to physiotherapists but it must be emphasised that it is artificial to separate and categorise the domains of human learning. There is considerable overlap and interdependency between the three areas.

PSYCHOMOTOR LEARNING

Motor skills are made up of abilities of which twenty have been identified by Fleishmann (1960, 1962, 1964) (Table 7.1). Abilites constitute the fundamental contituents of motor skills. An ability can be likened to an ingredient in a recipe where the motor skill would constitute the completed dish. An ability, therefore, can be defined as 'a general trait or capacity of an individual that is related to the performance of a variety of motor skills by being a component of those skills' structure' (Magill, 1980).

The term skill also has specific meaning in motor learning. Implied strongly in the use of the term is that it must be learned through appropriate practice. Skills, therefore, in terms of motor skills acquisition, can be defined as 'acts or tasks that require movement and must be learned in order to be properly performed' (Magill, 1980).

A skill is not an inherent characteristic. It must be acquired or learned through appropriate practice (Singer, 1972)

Skills are not all alike and it is useful to provide a framework which will allow classification and analysis (Fig. 7.1). It is possible

Table 7.1 Fundamental abilities of skilled performance (from Fleishman, 1960, 1962 &1964)

Psychomotor factors (11)
    Control precision
    Multilimb co-ordination
    Response orientation
    Reaction time
    Speed of arm movement
    Rate control
    Manual dexterity
    Finger dexterity
    Arm—hand steadiness
    Wrist finger speed
    Aiming

Physical proficiency (9)
    Extent flexibility
    Dynamic flexibility
    Explosive strength
    Static strength
    Dynamic strength
    Trunk strength
    Gross body co-ordination
    Gross body equilibrium
    Stamina

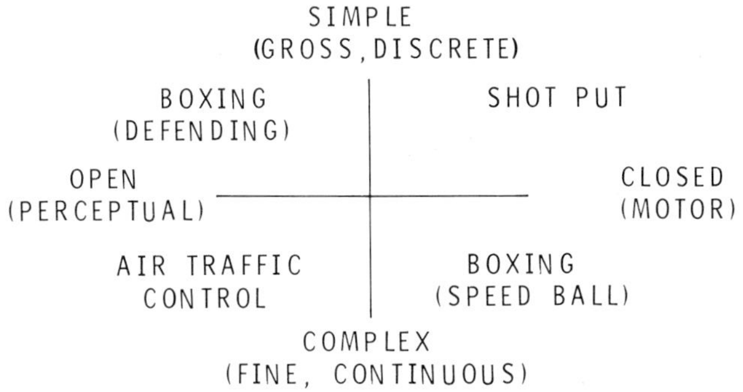

SIMPLE
(GROSS, DISCRETE)

BOXING
(DEFENDING)   SHOT PUT

OPEN   CLOSED
(PERCEPTUAL)   (MOTOR)

AIR TRAFFIC   BOXING
CONTROL   (SPEED BALL)

COMPLEX
(FINE, CONTINUOUS)

Fig. 7.1 Classification of skilled tasks (adapted from Holding, 1981)

to make distinctions between skills which mainly have perceptual demands, such as radar watch-keeping, and those which are predominantly motor, such as weight lifting. Along similar lines there are the closed skills which are executed with no reference to the environment—shot putting is an example—and the open skills which require a great deal of interaction with the environment, an example of which is kicking a moving soccer ball. Similarly, skills can have a distinct starting and finishing point and are referred to as discrete skills—pressing a button is a discrete skill. Conversely, skills which are on-going, such as turning a steering wheel of a car, are referred to as continuous skills. Skills can also be classified in terms of their magnitude. Gross skills usually involve whole body movements while fine skills are often complex, involving manual dexterity. The purpose of classifying skills is to facilitate description and analysis and permit the designing of appropriate learning modules and programmes ensuring the acquisition of a skill under optimum learning conditions.

THE PROCESS OF MOTOR SKILL ACQUISITION

Fitts, in 1964, described the process of motor learning as having three distinctive stages. In the cognitive phase the learner is made aware of the objectives and general principles of the task to be learned. It is thought that the conceptualisation of the skill requirements during this phase play an important role in motor learning and the phase can last from a few minutes to several hours depending upon the complexity of the task.

Following the cognitive phase, the learner then passes into the next phase of learning which is referred to as the fixation phase. Through continuous practice and repetition, motor behaviour is continually reorganised and the skill is gradually integrated into the mental set of the learner, the basis of which has been laid down in the cognitive phase. Extraneous movements are progressively eliminated and errors of movement and timing are reduced. The length of time of the fixation phase varies with the complexity of the task to be learned and the nature of the abilities of the learner but can last from several weeks to years.

The automatic phase is highlighted by the achievement of finely co-ordinated execution of the skill. The cognitive requirements of the learned task are reduced to a minimum allowing the learner to divert attention to other aspects of performance. The skill can be carried out under more demanding and complex conditions.

It should be pointed out that deterioration in performance can occur even after the automatic phase has been reached. These circumstances would necessitate a return to the earlier cognitive and fixation stages of skill acquisition in order to rectify the components of the skill which have been identified as the cause of the break-down in performance.

HUMAN INFORMATION PROCESSING (HIP)

Traditionally, physiotherapists have tended to develop and justify techniques of treatment in the neurosciences area using a neurophysiological framework (Brunnstrom, 1970; Bishop, 1982). Recently, the use of a human information processing model has been presented by Marteniuk (1979) and is an interesting alternative in the understanding and the re-education of disorders of function. In basic terms, the production of movement can be viewed as consisting of four fundamental components (Marteniuk, 1979). As shown in Figure 7.2, sensory input can be represented as an input mechanism with the CNS as a decision-making and processing unit. Appropriate output is effected by the contraction of muscle and the movement at joints and determination of the success of the output in achieving the objective is determined by a feedback mechanism. It can be seen that the appropriateness of movement can be affected by discrepencies in any of the four systems shown in this model. The same thing can be presented in neurophysiological terminology (Fig. 7.3). A more complex human information-processing framework permits much more detailed analysis of the factors which are required to deal successfully with information and create learning of movements which will result in mastery over a given task. The six-unit model presented by Sage (1977) and shown in Figure 7.4 deals with the reception of stimuli, attention to the information being received, perception, translation, the control of motor programmes, and the response behaviour. Several feedback systems are also integral components.

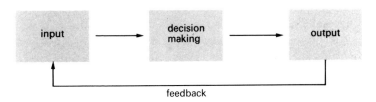

Fig. 7.2 Simple information processing model (from Sage G H 1977 Introduction to motor behaviour: A neuropsychological approach. Copyright 1977 Addison-Wesley. Reprinted by permission).

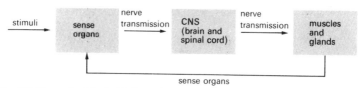

Fig. 7.3 Neurophysiological information processing model (from Sage G H 1977 Introduction to motor behaviour: A neuropsychological approach. Copyright 1977 Addison-Wesley. Reprinted by permission).

Reception of stimuli

Information which is required to permit the initiation of a skilled activity, enters the system by way of sensory input to the processing organism. This information, according to Holding (1965), informs the learner with regard to the nature of the task, the task itself and the monitoring of its accomplishment. Stimuli can be further subdivided into those which are generated externally and those which have an internal source. External stimuli provide the learner with information about the surrounding environment while internally generated stimuli occur largely as a result of discharge of receptors monitoring the function of muscle, joints, glands and other internal structures. A further category of stimulation is generated by the organism through cognition and thought processes (Sage, 1977).

In the early stages of skill acquisition it has been proposed that the learner relies heavily on visual sensory information (Fleishmen & Rich, 1963). With practice, however, control shifts from total reliance on vision to information supplied about the nature of the patterns of movement through periodic visual feedback (Pew, 1966) and an increased role of proprioception (Sage, 1977).

Selective attention

Clearly, it would be an impossible task for an individual to utilise all the information immediately available. Therefore, a selection of the pieces of information most useful to the successful accomplishment of the task is performed (Marteniuk, 1979). Selective attention deals with the way cues or messages are selected from the environment while others, less relevant, are ignored (Magill, 1980). The same author has referred to this concept as the 'cocktail party phenomenon', where the principle of the process is demonstrated when two people are engaged in conversation in a noisy environment. Extraneous noise is ignored, thus allowing the listener to hear

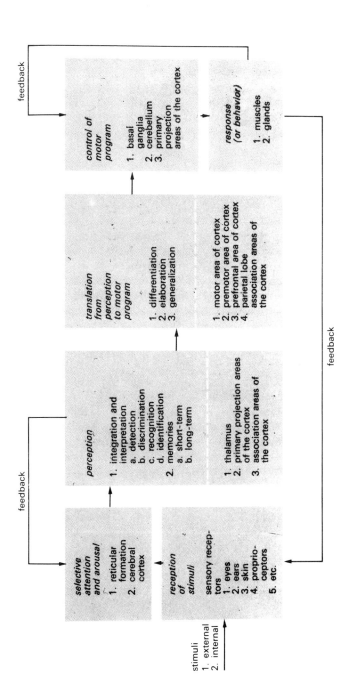

Fig. 7.4 Human information processing model (from Sage G H 1977 Introduction to motor behaviour: A neuropsychological approach. Copyright 1977 Addison-Wesley. Reprinted by permission).

and appreciate what is ignored, thus allowing the listener to hear and appreciate what the speaker is saying. It must be pointed out that this process of selective attention has a limited capacity. A number of studies have shown that an individual can only selectively attend to one source of information at one time (Cherry, 1953; Norman, 1968). In the learning of a new movement or task, selectively attending to only relevant pieces of information is built up by the learner through practice (Sage, 1977). When the execution of the task reaches a sophisticated level, the automatic phase described earlier, the performance of the task requires much less attention and the learner is then free to direct more attention to other facets of performance (Fitts, 1964).

Perception

Once sensory stimuli have been attended to, sense is made of them through processes of perception. This is the mechanism by which sensory information is obtained about the task, organised, integrated and interpreted to produce meaning (Sage, 1977). Figure 7.5 illustrates a common example of the function of this process. The picture can be interpreted in two ways by the observer, despite the fact that the source of visual information remains the same. Depending upon how the visual information is used, the reader will see either one piece of cake remaining or one piece removed.

The most basic of the perceptual tasks is detection which occurs when the individual can react when a predetermined stimulus has

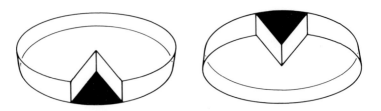

Fig. 7.5 Perceptual processes.

occurred. As this faculty develops, the learner is able to identify subtle properties previously missed. Detection becomes more sensitive and precise, and background irrelevant 'noise' is ignored (Fitts & Posner, 1967).

As perception develops, the learner is able to perform a discrimination between two very similar stimuli. An example of this can be seen in the sport of cricket where the batsman is able to discriminate between an off-break and a leg-break from the action of the bowler's arm. To the average viewer, both actions look identical unless observed repeatedly in slow motion with the subtle differences pointed out by an expert.

Higher order perceptual traits include recognition, the recall of familiar events, and identification where the performer can generate an appropriate response based upon minimal information (Fitts & Posner, 1967).

In motor skill acquisition all of these processes of perception become finely tuned and provide the learner with progressively more useful information. Perception relies heavily on the comparison of current information and previous experience. Therefore memory is also of fundamental importance (Sage, 1977).

Translation

Translation, as described by Sage (1977), refers to the process which links the perception of series of events to the initiation of an appropriate motor response. During this phase a motor programme consistent with the objective at hand is triggered and executed. Bartlett in 1932 stated 'when I make the (tennis) stroke I do not, as a matter of fact, produce something absolutely new and I never merely repeat something old'. Implicit in this statement is the concept that the motor response is not stereotyped and is tailored to meet the needs of the moment. Any sportsman who strives for consistency of performance can testify to the difficulty of producing the identical response on repeated occasions. It is thought by Schmidt (1975) that the basic sensory engram of the movement is 'set off' during this translation process. A tailor-made movement plan is then constructed utilising all available and current information of environmental conditions. With practice the translation process becomes more specific resulting in more appropriate responses.

The development of motor programmes is thought to follow a process similar to the hierarchical learning of cognitive function as described by Bloom et al (1956) through a process of differentiation, elaboration and generalisation (Sage, 1977).

Differentiation describes the initial process of sorting complimentary movement components together. Random movement, which is characteristic of the newborn, is replaced by the appearance of more sophisticated patterns of movement, and extraneous, irrelevant movement is eliminated. Godfrey and Kephart (1969) have defined a movement pattern as an 'extensive group or series of motor acts which are performed with lesser degrees of skill (than a motor skill) but which are directed toward accomplishment of some external purpose.' Magill (1980) has defined the movement pattern as a basic component of movement that can be generalised to the specific demands of a particular motor skill.

Differentiation is followed by elaboration, where the learner experiments by producing varying motor responses, all of which are attempts to attain the same objective. Finally, the learner begins to generalise the already developed motor programmes to similar but novel tasks. An example of this is seen when an individual who is an accomplished tennis player generalises the tennis strokes to squash, although he may never have played the latter racket sport before. As a consequence, the skill of the individual in both sports may suffer.

It should be noted that the concepts described above as characteristic of the translation process are consistent with the notion of patterns of movement elaborated by Knott and Voss (1967) as a fundamental component of the PNF approach to therapeutic exercise.

Motor program control

In terms of the acquisition of a given motor skill, it has been proposed by Adams (1971) that the learner utilises a memory trace which serves to select and execute a response which, initially, will be somewhat crude in quality of precision. As the individual receives feedback information concerning the appropriateness of the response, the perceptual trace begins to form which becomes the image against which all future responses specific to the task being learned are compared. With practice the movement generated becomes more efficient in achieving the criterion task and the perceptual trace strengthens leading to further refinements in performance. Control becomes less dependent upon visual feedback mechanisms and the role of proprioceptive feedback becomes more pronounced.

A number of researchers have suggested the presence of two feedback systems both of which are important in the control and subsequent modification of motor responses—a long-term loop and a short-term loop (Schmidt, 1975; Magill, 1980; Schmidt & McCabe, 1976). The long-term feedback takes approximately 200 milliseconds to effect a movement modification and utilises visual, auditory and proprioceptive information. The purpose of this feedback system is to issue a new series of instructions to the motor programme (Welford, 1968). The short loop takes a much shorter period of time, approximately 30 milliseconds, to modify movement and does not entail the issuing of new instructions to the motor programme. It is thought that the purpose of the short loop is to influence and make discrete corrections to the individual components of movement on a continuous and on-going basis throughout the execution of the movement. It is believed that this short loop feedback system is centrally located (Sage, 1977).

Feedback

A vital element in the eventual construction of finely tuned movement is the important role of feedback. Feedback serves to detect errors in the execution of the performance which leads to attempts by the learner to reduce error.

Feedback, from a motor learning viewpoint, can be described in terms of knowledge of performance (KP) and knowledge of results (KR). KP has been described by Marteniuk (1979) as the feedback received by an individual about the execution of the actual performance of a skill. This type of feedback is generated from the variety of sources of proprioceptive information. Feedback, in the form of KR, has been described by Bilodeau and Bilodeau (1961) as the single most important variable influencing skill acquisition and it has been proposed by Adams (1978) as a major source of intrinsic motivation to the learner. KR is usually generated from an external source and provides information to the learner concerning the success of the movement in achieving the objective of the movement. In soccer, for example, the person shooting the ball receives KR when the ball hits or misses the goal.

It can be seen from examination of the HIP model that there are many important factors which must be taken into account when considering both the production of movement skills and their acquisition. A disorder of movement can arise as a result of abnormal functioning in any part of the systems described and the HIP model is useful in conceptualising and analysing the effect of disturbances in the component parts (Turnbull, 1983).

MECHANISMS OF RECOVERY FOLLOWING CNS DAMAGE

Recovery of function following CNS damage is thought to be brought about by two basic mechanisms (Yu, 1980). Re-organisation theory proposes that recovery occurs by means of morphological adjustment of undamaged neural circuitry which results in permanent changes in the function of those neurons. Conversely, the re-establishment theory asserts that recovery takes place as a result of sparing of some or all of the neural mechanisms which mediated the activity before the damage. A further possibility is that both processes may contribute.

The processes which utilise these mechanisms have been listed as shown in Table 7.2, but it remains unclear which mechanism predominates or whether all contribute. Regardless of this, it seems reasonable to assume that physiotherapy is attempting to influence this recovery process, particularly equipotentiality, redundancy and behaviour substitution. In addition, Bach-y-Rita (1981) has proposed that environmental factors and consideration of learning theory are two further areas which need investigation as influences on the recovery process in stroke, and both of these areas are fundamental to the provision of physiotherapy.

Table 7.2   Possible mechanisms of CNS recovery with training

1. SPROUTING
2. DENERVATION SUPERSENSITIVITY
3. DISAPPEARANCE OF SHOCK
4. EQUIPOTENTIALITY
5. REDUNDANCY
6. BEHAVIOUR SUBSTITUTION

THE IMPLICATIONS OF COMPONENT DISORDER OF THE H.I.P. MODEL TO PHYSIOTHERAPY IN THE MANAGEMENT OF STROKE

Stroke can result in a wide variety of symptoms and can include altered sensation, diminished attention span, deficiencies of memory, disorders of perception and alterations of motor function (Adams, 1974). Any one or a variety of combinations of those symptoms can significantly alter the learning and production of movement for reasons which become clear when the HIP model is examined. It is important to recognise that disorders of functional movement can result from abnormalities in systems other than the effector motor system. In fact, Rout (1978) has proposed that the pure motor stroke is a rare occurrence. Therefore, in order to maximise functional recovery through therapeutic exercise, the physiotherapist would be wise to consider the possible effects on movement production of disordered function of each component of the HIP model.

Disorders of reception of stimuli

Diminished sensation, particularly proprioceptive and visual, would theoretically compromise the ability of the stroke patient to obtain environmental information and to monitor the function of limb components as movement is executed with a consequent effect on appropriate movement production. Aberrant sensation produced by such clinical manifestations as visual field deficit may result in abormal movement responses due to the important role of vision in the early stages of skill acquisition. Similarly, diminished proprioceptive sense may require augmentation through some form of feedback enhancement (e.g. joint position biofeedback, mirrors or specific sensory cueing by the physiotherapist) before desired learning will occur. It must be also be recognized that the frequent repetition of abnormal movement will create, within the patient, a learned sensory association. This would most likely result in the consolidation of the production of abnormal movement, and emphasises the proposal made by several authors that abnormal movement must be inhibited at all times (Bobath, 1970; Todd, 1974), particularly in the early stages post stroke (Dardier, 1980; Turnbull & Bell, 1983).

Patient-generated internal stimuli may also be deficient, with a consequent effect on movement production. Adams (1974) and Bogardh and Richards (1981) have suggested that an important factor which interferes with the re-education of movement may be the inability of the patient to learn due to disruption of higher cognitive function. These assertions would seem to be feasible based on the role of internally generated stimuli in the HIP model.

Disorders of selective attention

The complex problems presented to physiotherapists by stroke patients with a 'diminished attention span' is well known to most clinicians. It is important that the attention of the patient is specifically directed towards key stimulus indicators, bearing in mind that the capacity of selective attention is limited even in a person with no neurological deficit. Treating stroke patients in a noisy physiotherapy gymnasium or in a busy ward in the early stages of recovery would seem to provide an impossible environment for the person with a diminished attention span. External stimuli should be controlled wherever possible so that the patient is not distracted away from the task at hand.

Patients who do not appear to have a reduced attention span should also be taught to attend to the key stimuli which are of most importance to the mastery of the task to be learned. In the words of Whiting 'one of the criteria on which a teacher (physiotherapist) might be judged successful is his ability to make his trainee's attention selective by pointing out toward what part of the display his perceptual systems need to be orientated and the information he is trying to abstract. Unsophisticated teachers (physiotherapists) may fail to appreciate that the beginner (patient) may not be utilising the same information as the expert (author's brackets).

Disorders of perception

Many authors, including Siev and Freishtat (1976) and Gartland and Woon (1981), have proposed that consideration of disorders of perception is of paramount importance in the motor re-education of some patients with stroke, particularly those with parietal and temporal lobe damage of the non-dominant hemisphere (Friedland & Weinstien 1978). Examination of the HIP model clearly shows that dysfunction of perception is likely to have a profound effect on motor activity. Attention, therefore, to the identification and remediation of these problems is necessary before motor performance will be improved to a significant degree. Ayres (1962) has proposed a number of remedial strategies to improve such disorders, but generally speaking perceptual disturbances tend to receive only cursory attention from physiotherapists. There has been a tendency, within rehabilitation teams, to delegate totally the responsibility for perceptual testing and treatment to occupational therapists and, more recently, neuropsychologists (Filskov & Boll,

1981). To cope effectively with the re-education of motor competencies, an understanding of the role of perception in the production of movement is essential.

In terms of motor re-education it would seem logical to re-educate perception in the hierarchical sequence presented in the HIP model, commencing with the ability to detect a predetermined stimulus through to the generation of responses based upon minimal information.

Perusal of physiotherapy literature clearly shows that little emphasis has been placed on the importance of perceptual processes in motor rehabilitation. The HIP model shows clearly that in movement generation and skills acquisition, perception is an important and fundamental ingredient. Therefore, attention to the role and remediation of perceptual deficit is of considerable importance in the rehabilitation of functional movement (Ruskin, 1982).

Disorders of translation

Any dysfunction of the translation process will manifest as an inability by the patient to trigger a motor programme which is consistent with the achievement of the desired objective. Ayres (1962) has referred to this process as sensory motor integration. It seems important that all three translation components are re-educated in the treatment of the stroke patient. For example, if the patient was unable to elaborate motor responses the result would be the generation of movement patterns which would be stereotyped and inappropriate to cope with the immediate demands of the presented task. Similarly, if the patient did not have the ability to generalise the motor programmes to similar but novel tasks, new situations would result in movements inaccuracies. In gait re-education, the patient must be capable of making adjustments to motor patterns learned in the gymnasium to cope with uneven surfaces, inclines and wet conditions. The ability to generalise is important to permit this adaptation.

Disorders of motor programme control

In order to produce a movement which satisfies the demands of the task being undertaken, it is necessary for the performer to possess, from a motor viewpoint, an image of the desired movement. If these conditions are not met, inappropriate movement will result. The long and short loop feedback systems will be unable to modify the movement to 'fit' that which is desirable, and movement errors in terms of accuracy and timing will be produced. In addition, if these feedback systems are deficient, modifications to the motor programme will not be made in the light of new information perceived by the system with a similar result. It is likely that the result will be in the form of a dysynergic ataxia.

Disorders of the feedback system

Inability to recognise and utilise feedback in the form of KR is likely to compromise seriously the learning process and all other attempts by the person to reduce errors in movement performance. It is important that the physiotherapist makes allowance within treatment sessions to ensure that the patient is provided with meaningful KR. This important topic will be discussed more fully later in this chapter.

THE APPLICATION OF SPECIFIC MOTOR SKILLS ACQUISITION THEORY TO THE MANAGEMENT OF THE STROKE PATIENT

As outlined earlier in the chapter, the acquisition of motor skills has been divided into cognitive, fixation and automatic phases by Fitts (1964). Although the supporting research basis generated from this area of study has been gleaned from populations with intact CNS, it would seem logical to assume that people with neurological deficit would benefit from the application of these principles. It should be pointed out that the use of motor learning theory should not be viewed as a replacement for the current physiotherapy approaches in the neurosciences, but rather as a body of knowledge which will enhance the effectiveness of these current techniques (Turnbull, 1982). The remainder of this paper will present specific items from the three phase model of skills acquisition of Fitts (1964) and discuss their application to the physiotherapy management of the stroke patient.

Cognitive issues

During this phase the learner develops an overall idea of the skill to be learned. This objective is achieved by the instructor who will describe the objectives and the nature of the activity, either by demonstration or by exposing the learner to the observation of the skill being performed by an expert often by means of a videotape. This process leads to the development by the learner of a task specific mental-set (Martenuik, 1979). During this phase of motor learning effective communication is an important measurement (Fitts & Posner, 1967).

The physiotherapist, in explaining the task to be learned to the patient, is identifying the objectives of the movement sequence. However, recently, in a study designed to teach crutch walking, Gonella et al (1981) found that the use of videotapes during the cognitive phase improved the quality of movement and the speed of learning when compared with conventional methods. These results tend to indicate that a similar procedure may well be successful in stroke management, particularly in the teaching of complex movements such as gait. This proposal is strengthened when consideration is given to the fact that instruction, currently, is provided by verbal means. It may well be that the use of additional communication mediums may be more effective, particularly if the patient exhibits disordered higher cortical function including language dysfunction.

Fixation issues

This phase of motor learning, which can last from a few weeks to several years, is characterised by regular periods of practice during which the learner continuously reorganises motor behaviour. Timing, speed and accuracy of movement patterns are refined, and complementary components of the skill are combined. Extraneous movements are gradually eliminated and co-ordination between independent movement constituents is developed. The learner attempts to reduce performance error with the result that, eventually, the criterion task can be accurately performed in a consistent manner (Robb, 1972).

In the management of the stroke patient the period of re-education can be regarded as the period of practice with the objective of the re-acquisition of functional competencies (Turnbull, 1983).

Practice

It has been shown quite conclusively that there is a positive correlation between practice and the improvement of task performance, measured as a reduction in the number of errors and shown in

Figure 7.6 (Trussell, 1965). It has also been demonstrated by Cross-mann (1959) that in some instances improvements in performance can continue for up to seven years, evidenced in the famous cigar-making study (Fig. 7.7). In stroke rehabilitation, treatment has been continued until the functional status appears stable, usually around 9 months post stroke at which time the emphasis on active treatment is reduced (Bach-y-Rita, 1981).The same author and Lane (1978) have questioned these traditional time frames, citing the growing evidence in the literature to suggest that recovery can continue for up to six years following the initial lesion. The implication of this proposal is that patients will require access to continuing therapeutic exercise if they are to attain and maintain full functional potential. For the reasons articulated by Lane (1978), innovative physiotherapy strategies will be required to ensure that people, recovering from stroke have the full opportunity to continue practice of activities designed to improve functional movement. This could possibly be achieved by the judicious use of close family members, whom Carr and Shepherd (1982) have referred to as 'an untapped resource', and to the use of current technology in the form of microcomputers (Turnbull, 1983).

Frequency of practice

The optimum frequency of physiotherapy, which would include the

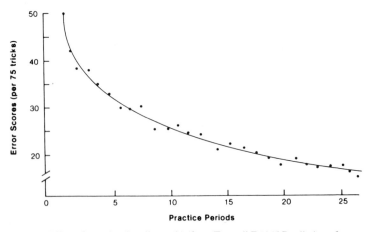

Fig. 7.6 Effect of practice (juggling task) (from Trussell E 1965 Prediction of success in a motor skill on the basis of early learning achievement. Research Quarterly 36: 342–347 (figure 1). Published by the American Alliance for Health, Physical Education, Recreation and Dance. Reprinted by permission).

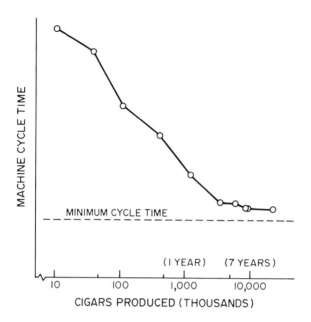

Fig. 7.7 Prolonged practice (adapted from Crossman, 1959).

practice of movement sequences, has not been determined. In most centres recent strokes are treated by physiotherapy at least once daily. However, when offered this suggestion by a student this author asked how many treatments a week this would mean; the response was five times a week because physiotherapists do not work at weekends. It has been proposed by Carr and Shepherd (1982) that the patient should be exposed to rehabilitation-derived procedures at times in addition to the period spent with the physiotherapist. Turnbull and Bell (1983) and Dardier (1980) have suggested procedures whereby appropriate movement patterns are encouraged and practised during routine nursing care. This wide exposure to therapeutic exercise is likely to have a more significant effect than practice which occurs only during formal physiotherapy sessions. It is clear, however, that the frequency of practice question requires an answer which will only be obtained through carefully controlled clinical research.

Content of practice

In the field of motor skills acquisition, distinctions are made between whole-practice, in which the whole skill is rehearsed, and part-practice, in which parts of the whole skill are practised prior to the complete task being constructed. It is often a difficult decision to decide how much of the skill can be attempted at any one time. In physiotherapy management it is common for a specific part of the movement to be practised independently, an example of which is the component procedures of the gait cycle as described by Bobath (1977). Procedures which are designed to transfer the centre of mass of the body through the involved lower limb, are practised first in the supine position and later in sitting. The resultant facilitation of equilibrium responses permits the patient to re-acquire the ability to balance on the affected leg, with the objective of improving the support phase of gait on the affected leg. The ultimate result of this regime is an improvement in gait symmetry (Wall & Ashburn, 1979). Examples of this process are shown in Figures 7.8–7.11.

In some instances it may be more effective to have the patient practise the whole skill. Singer (1980) has presented a framework

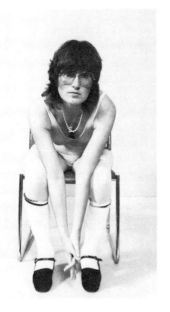

Fig. 7.8 Procedure to encourage symmetrical weight-transfer through both lower limbs

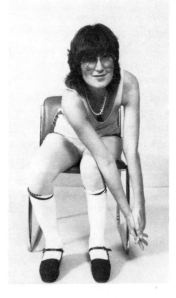

Fig. 7.9 Part-practice of support phase of gait of affected leg

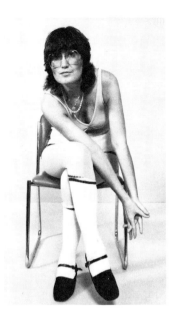

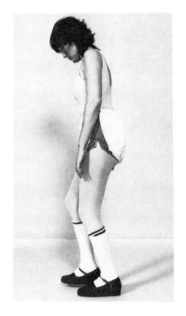

Fig. 7.10 Part-practice of support phase. Patient shifts centre of mass over affected leg

Fig. 7.11 Whole-practice of support phase of gait on affected side

to assist in deciding which method is more successful. In Figure 7.12 two continua are presented, dealing with task organisation and task complexity. A task is said to be highly organised when the components are intimately related to each other. Where the components are relatively independent the task exhibits low organisation (Magill, 1980). Task complexity refers to the number of components which constitute the task and the accompaning attention demands. It can be seen in Figure 12 that where tasks exhibit high task organisation but low task complexity levels, the whole-method has been found to be more effective as a learning paradigm than part-methods in people with normal CNS. In tasks which are both high in organisation and complexity a combination of whole- and part-methods are indicated. In the world of sport, for example, a cover drive in cricket demands a great deal of attention and consists of many components which would place it high in terms of task complexity. The components, however, vary in their inter-relationship with each other in terms of their dependence. The back swing is relatively distinct from the forward part of the stroke. The

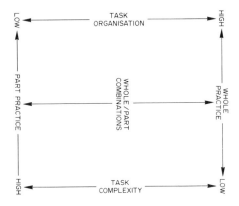

Fig. 7.12 Task organisation and task complexity (adapted from Singer, 1980).

high complexity of this stroke would tend to favour the practice of large combinations of the total shot while the intermediate level of task organisation would suggest a combination of whole- and part-practice. The decision based on these two considerations would probably result in the utilisation of a modified part-practice, where certain dependent component sequences would be practised together while more independent components would be practised separately. With reference to the recovering stroke patients, even simple movements are attention demanding, which automatically raises the level of task complexity and strongly suggests part-practice perhaps at the most basic component level. However, as the patient acquires the movement and the attention demands of the task reduce, consideration should be given to the level of organisation of the task. The support phase on the swing phase of gait can be considered to have a high level of task organisation. Therefore, these components will probably be more successfully acquired if practised in more of a whole-method manner. However, the decision should be viewed not as a choice between whole- or part-methods but rather in terms of degrees along the continuum for each consideration.

Knowledge of results

KR provides information to the learner about the success of the movement which has just been executed. All theories of skills acquisition cite this factor as of major importance (Thorndike, 1927; Schmidt, 1982). Figure 7.13 shows the effect of different KR

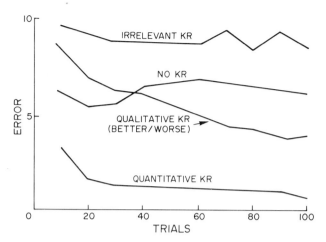

Fig. 7.13 Effects of different KR on error reduction (adapted from Trowbridge and Carson, 1932)

conditions on the learning of a task. It can be seen that both irrelevant KR and no KR did not result in any learning. This finding underscores the significant importance of this learning variable. In the same Figure, quantitative KR can be seen to be more effective in promoting learning than qualitative (Better/Worse) KR. Physiotherapists typically provide KR, subjectively the relevance, accuracy and consistency of which is dependent upon the experience of the clinician (Wall & Ashburn, 1979). Efforts should be made to provide the patient with more meaningful quantitative KR to enhance the learning of specific functional tasks. The success of biofeedback can perhaps be explained by the ability of the modality to provide the patient with consistent, accurate and quantitative KR.

Mirrors have been used for some time now in the treatment of stroke to provide the patient with visual feedback of their performance as attempts are made to re-acquire symmetrical sitting balance. Theoretically, this procedure is sound in that vision is heavily utilised in the early part of the learning process (Newell, 1973). However, it should be ascertained that the patient can perceive and adjust to the reversal of the mirror image. The use of mirrors may be made more effective by the placing of patient-specific reference lines on the mirror perhaps to identify clearly the mid-line of the body and to indicate the level of the shoulders. This strategy would provide the patient with more information, rendering the KR from the mirror more specific and therefore enhancing learning. Similarly, advances in technology, such as microcomputers and videotapes, should be monitored by physiotherapists in efforts to develop devices which will provide specific quantitative feedback.

It must also be recognised that manipulating KR will have an effect on the process of skill re-acquisition. Providing the patient with positive feedback to maintain or improve the morale of the patient will adversely affect movement re-education (Turnbull, 1982). Similarly, KR should be given for one aspect of the skill at a time due to the limited capacity of attention mechanisms and to prevent interference. Shea & Upton (1976) showed that when a motor activity was introduced into the period immediately following the completion of a skill acquisition trial and before the provision of KR, the KR-delay interval, the learning of the skill was adversely affected (Fig. 7.14). This finding would seem to be important in stroke management, particularly in cases where memory has been affected. A further justification for physiotherapists to attempt to improve provision of KR is the influence of this variable upon motivation. Adams (1978) has proposed that error reduction is a powerful intrinsic motivator. Before an individual can reduce error, the magnitude and the direction of the error must be apparent. The presentation of specific KR will provide this error information and it is likely that motivation will be maintained. This is an important consideration, given that the therapeutic exercise may be provided to stroke patients for several years in the future, thereby presenting the further problem of patient compliance.

The learning environment

It has been shown clearly that environmental conditions influence the CNS both behaviourally and morphologically (Walsh & Greenough, 1976). This would seem to be applicable in the management of the stroke patient. Careful attention to constructing the environment on the affected side of the patient is an important consideration, particularly in the acute-care ward setting (Turnbull & Bell, 1983). The purpose of this strategy is to stimulate the attention of the patient toward the hemiplegic side, thus encouraging body symmetry. Similarly, it is important that a contribution is made by the patient in all routine nursing care activities to prevent the appearance of learned non-use. In a study described by Yu (1980), monkeys, with a surgically induced hemiplegia, were found to use the affected hand for feeding several days post-stroke when the non-

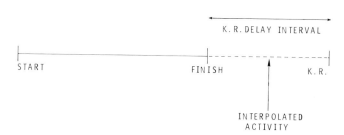

Fig. 7.14 Interpolated activity in the KR delay interval (based on Shea and Upton, 1978)

affected hand was restrained. A control group of similar animals quickly compensated for the functional loss by using the non-affected upper extremity while the affected limb was not used at all. This finding would tend to suggest that learned non-use of the involved extremity readily occurs and further supports the assertions of Bobath (1977) towards stimulating the affected side. It is likely that attention to environmental factors is an important consideration in stroke rehabilitation.

Automatic phase issues

In this phase of learning the learner is able to perform the acquired task in a highly efficient manner under complex and demanding conditions (Fitts, 1964). The performer is able to concentrate on other attention-demanding items while the learned skill is being executed at a high level of efficiency. This phenomenon can be observed in driving a car. Initially, the learner must devote full attention to observing the rules of the road and operating the vehicle. In the early stages these endeavours demand the full attention of the driver. As learning progresses, the more experienced driver is able to drive the car safely while enjoying the scenery and conversing with a passenger. Similarly, the person learning a skill is only able, in the early stages of skill acquisition, to concentrate on the specifics of the task. Later, the learner can attend to strategy and elaboration of the task as the skill integration enters the automatic phase.

In stroke rehabilitation, the patient initially must concentrate fully on the exercises, such as practice of the individual components of the gait cycle. The objective of treatment, however, must be to re-educate the walking pattern to the extent that the patient is able to walk while attentding to other factors. An example of this occurs when the patient wishes to cross a busy intersection. The patient should be able to walk across the road with attention being paid to the potential hazards posed by approaching automobiles rather than concentrating on the components of gait. It is well known by physiotherapists that the performance of patients who walk well in the gymnasium, often deteriorates when the patient leaves the department, probably because the demands of coping with the environment diverts attention away from gait. It could be proposed that the patient has not yet reached the automatic phase of gait and that further practice with KR is required. If the patient is discharged from treatment before the automatic phase is reached, the constant attention demands of the patient to other areas may exacerbate a deterioration in performance with the subsequent development and entrenchment of abnormal movement patterns. This would require a return to both the cognitive and fixation phases of skill acquisition, with accompanying social and economic ramifications. It seems important that the everyday activity competencies are relearned to the automatic stage so that movement becomes an automatic consideration to the stroke person rather than an item that demands a great deal of attention.

Although gait relearning has been used as the example in this section, the same principles apply to all functional movement competencies re-educated in the physiotherapy department.

CONCLUSION

The purpose of this chapter was the presentation and application, to stroke rehabilitation, of some principles and theory from the field of motor skills acquisition. The major assumption of this perspective is that the processes known to influence the recovery of function following CNS damage are influenced by the experiences to which the patient is exposed during physical treatment. Bach-y-Rita (1981) has proposed that learning theory is a potentially useful avenue to investigate as a method of maximising the re-education of function in stroke. The same author has suggested that the stroke patient may reach a number of performance plateaus throughout the duration of the reacquisition process. Following the reaching of automatic phases in a number of movements, the patient is then in a position to cope with additional information-processing demands which is accompanied with further improvement. This process is both dynamic and on-going and may continue over several years, thereby strongly suggesting the need for non-traditional and innovative physiotherapy delivery methods. This may require that the accepted role of the physiotherapist, in this continuing care area, will require re-evaluation. More emphasis would likely be placed on assessment, review, teaching of relatives who will be responsible for the supervision of the exercises on a day-to-day basis, home-based programmes and the development of computer-feedback technology to overcome problems of compliance.

The application of a skills acquisition model in the management of stroke, in addition to improving current physiotherapy management models, may also provide a useful research paradigm. The problem of the lack of evaluation in physiotherapy has been well documented and is a most difficult area, particularly in the area of stroke rehabilitation. Modification of significant research in the motor learning area would permit investigators to draw comparisons between healthy populations and those disabled by stroke. This endeavour would result in a clearer understanding of the learning conditions which would be optimal in stroke management, thus improving physiotherapy care in this area.

It must be made explicitly clear that the proposals presented in this chapter are largely unconfirmed in their application to stroke management. This is not unusual in physiotherapy. However, it is of vital importance that such theories are tested rigorously and systematically by physiotherapists before any dramatic claims are made. The need for research in physiotherapy is of paramount importance to the development and maintenance of a viable professional body of knowledge and for the ultimate objective of improving patient care.

REFERENCES

Adams G F 1974 Cerebrovascular disease and the ageing brain. Churchill Livingstone, Edinburgh
Adams J A 1971 A closed-loop theory of motor learning. Journal of Motor Behaviour 5: 111–150
Adams J A 1978 Theoretical issues of knowledge of results. In: Stelmach G E (ed) Information processing in motor control and learning. Academic Press, New York
Andrews K, Brocklehurst J C, Richards B, Laycock P J 1980 The prognostic value of picture drawings by stroke patients. Rheumatology and Rehabilitation 19: 180–188
Atkinson H W 1982 Principles of treatment. In: Downie P A (ed) Cash's textbook of neurology for physiotherapists. Faber and Faber, London

Ayres J A 1962 Perception of space of adult hemiplegic patients. Archives of Physical Medicine 43: 552–555

Bach-y-Rita P 1981 Brain plasticity as a basis of the development of rehabilitation procedures for hemiplegia. Scandinavian Journal of Rehabilitation Medicine 13: 73–83

Bartlett F 1932 Remembering. Cambridge University Press, Cambridge

Bilodeau E A, Bilodeau I M 1961 Motor skills learning. Annual Review of Psychology 12: 243–280

Bishop B 1982 Basic neurophysiology. Medical Examination Publishing Company, Garden City

Bloom B S 1956 Taxonomy of educational objectives, handbook 1: cognitive domain. McKay, New York

Bobath B 1970 Adult hemiplegia: evaluation and treatment. Heinemann, London

Bobath B 1977 Evaluation and management of adult hemiplegia. Heinemann, London

Bogardh E, Richards C L 1981 Gait analysis and relearning of gait control in hemiplegic patients. Physiotherapy Canada 33: 223–230

Brocklehurst J C, Andrews K, Richards B, Laycock P J 1978 How much physical therapy for patients with stroke? British Medical Journal 1 (6123): 1307–1310

Brunnstrom S 1970 Movement therapy in hemiplegia. Harper and Row, London

Carr J H, Shepherd R B 1980 Physiotherapy in disorders of the brain. Heinemann, London

Carr J H, Shepherd R B 1983 A motor relearning programme for stroke. Aspen, Rockville, Maryland and Heinemann, London

Cherry C 1953 Some experiments on the recognition of speech with one and with two ears. Journal of the Acoustical Society of America 25: 975–979

Crossman E R F 1959 A theory of the acquisition of speed skill. Ergonomics 2: 153–166

Dardier E 1980 The early stroke patient: positioning and movment. Bailliere Tindall, London

Filskov S B, Boll T J (eds) 1981 Handbook of clinical neuropsychology. Wiley, New York

Fitts P M 1964 Perceptual motor learning skill. In: Melton A W (ed) Categories of human learning. Academic Press, New York

Fitts P M, Posner M I 1967 Human performance. Brooks and Cole, Belmont, California

Fleishman E A 1960 Psychomotor tests in drug research. In: Miller J G, Uhr L (eds) Drugs and behaviour. Wiley, New York

Fleishman E A 1962 The description and prediction of perceptual-motor skill learning. In: Gaser R (ed) Training research and education. University of Pittsburgh Press, Pittsburgh

Fleishman E A 1964 The structure and measurement of physical fitness. Prentice Hall, New Jersey

Fleishman E A, Rich S 1963 Role of kinaesthetic and spatial-visual abilities in perceptual-motor learning. Journal of Experimental Psychology 66: 6–11

Friedland R P, Weinsten E A 1977 Hemi-inattention and hemisphere specialisation. Introduction and historical review. In: Weinstein E A, Friedland (eds) Advances in neurology volume 18. Raven Press, New York.

Gartland G J, Woon L H 1981 Testing and treatment for some sensory defects in stroke rehabilitation. Physiotherapy Canada 33: 347–354

Godfrey B B, Kephart N C 1969 Movement patterns and motor education. Appleton-Century-Crofts, New York

Gonnella C, Kalish R, Hale G. 1978 A commentary on electromyographic feedback in physical therapy. Physical Therapy 58: 11–14

Gonnella C, Hale G, Ionta M, Perry J C 1981 Self-instruction in a perceptual motor skill. Physical Therapy 61: 177–184

Holding D H 1981 Skills research. In: Holding D H (ed) Human skills. Wiley, Toronto

Isaacs B 1978 Problems and solutions in rehabilitating stroke patients. Geriatrics 33: 87–91

Knott M, Voss D 1968 Proprioceptive neuromuscular facilitation—patterns and techniques. Harper and Row, New York

Krathwohl D R, Bloom B S, Masia B R 1964 Taxonomy of educational objectives, handbook 2: affective domain. McKay, New York

Lane R E J 1978 Facilitation of weight transference in the stroke patient. Physiotherapy 64: 260–264

Magill R A 1980 Motor learning concepts and applications. Brown, Dubeqe, Iowa

Marteniuk R G 1979 Motor skill performance and learning: considerations for rehabilitation. Physiotherapy Canada 31: 187–202

McCann C, Culbertson R 1976 Comparison of two systems for stroke rehabilitation in a general hospital. Journal of the American Geriatric Society 24: 211–216

Norman D A 1968 Toward a theory of memory and attention. Psychological Review 75: 522–536

Pew R W 1966 Acquisition of hierarchical control over the temporal organisation of a skill. Journal of Experimental Psychology 71: 764–771

Pryse-Phillips W, Murray T J 1982 Essential neurology, Medical Examination Publication Co Inc, New York

Redford J B, Harris J D 1980 Rehabilitation of the elderly stroke patient. American Family Physician 22:

Robb M D 1972 Man in sports: the acquisition of skill. In: Christina R W, Shaver L G (eds) Biological and psychological perspectives in the study of human behaviour. Kendall/Hurst, Dubeque, Iowa

Rout M W 1978 Disorders of perception in stroke. Age and Aging 7: 22–36

Ruskin A P 1982 Understanding stroke and its rehabilitation. Current Concepts of Cerebrovascular Disease Stroke 17: 27–32

Sage G H 1977 Introduction to motor behaviour: A neuropsychological approach. Addison-Wesley, Reading, Massachusetts

Schmidt R A 1975 A schema theory of discrete motor skill learning. Psychological Review 82: 225–260

Schmidt R A 1982 Motor control and learning. Human Kinetics, Champagne, Illinois

Schmidt R A, McCabe J F 1976 Motor program utilization over extended practice. Journal of Human Movement Studies 2: 239–247

Shea J B, Upton G 1978 The effects on skill acquisition of an interpolated motor short term memory task during the KR delay interval. Journal of Motor Behavior 8: 277–281

Siev E, Freishtat B 1976 Perceptual dysfunction in the adult stroke patient. A manual for evaluation and treatment. Charles B. Slack, New York

Singer R N 1972 Readings in motor learning. Lea and Febiger, Philadelphia

Singer R N 1980 Motor learning and human performance, 3rd edn. Macmillan, New York.

Stockmeyer S A 1967 An interpretation of the approach of Rood to the treatment of neuromuscular dysfunction. American Journal of Physical Medicine 46: 900–956

Stonnington H 1980 Rehabilitation in cerebrovascular diseases. In: Royden Janes H (ed) Primary care: clinics in office practice, Saunders, Toronto

Thorndike E L 1927 Law of effect. American Journal of Psychology 16: 212–222

Todd J 1974 Physiotherapy in the early stages of hemiplegia. Physiotherapy 60: 336–342

Trussell E 1965 Prediction of success in a motor skill on the basis of early learning achievement. Research Quarterly 36: 342–347

Turnbull G I 1982 Some learning theory implications in neurological physiotherapy. Physiotherapy 68: 38–41

Turnbull G I 1983 Learning psychology in neurological physiotherapy. Unpublished Presentation, Annual Congress of the Canadian Physiotherapy Association, Winnipeg, Manitoba

Turnbull G I, Bell P A 1983 Recovery maximised: nursing the acute stroke patient to maximize functional recovery. Nova Scotia Heart Foundation, Halifax, Nova Scotia

Voss D E 1967 Proprioceptive neuromuscular facilitation. American Journal of Physical Medicine 46: 838–898

Wall J C, Ashburn A 1979 Assessment of gait disability in hemiplegics. Scandinavian Journal of Rehabilitation Medicine 11: 95–103

Walsh R N, Greenough W T (eds) 1976 Environments as therapy for brain dysfunction. Plenum Press, New York

Welford A T 1968 Fundamentals of skill. Methuen, London

Whiting H T A 1972 Overview of the skill learning process. Research Quarterly 43: 266–294

Yu J 1980 Neuromuscular recovery with training after central nervous system lesions: an experimental approach. In: Ince L P (ed) Behavioural psychology in rehabilitation medicine: clinical applications. Williams and Wilkins, Baltimore

Educational programmes for those involved in the total care of the stroke patient

INTRODUCTION

There are several factors which affect the quality and outcome of rehabilitation. During the last three decades physical therapists have, in trying to improve the quality of rehabilitation, focused their attention on what is happening in individual therapy sessions.

A lot of time has been spent in developing the physical therapist's own manual skill in techniques based upon neurophysiological approaches (Brunnstrom, 1970; Bobath, 1978). In spite of having well trained physical therapists at hand, many stroke patients fail to reach the rehabilitation goals set up for them. This fact drew our attention to what was happening to the patient outside the therapy session. We found that the patient was subjected to different and contradictory methods of rehabilitation from nursing staff, different paramedical professions and relatives. We drew the conclusion that one of the most important factors affecting the quality of rehabilitation has to be the consistency of methods and goals. We also found that the nursing staff often had a pessimistic attitude towards the stroke patient's potential for recovery. This probably has a negative impact on the patient's motivation and, accordingly, may be another reason for poor rehabilitation results. A project for patients with stroke was started in 1977 at Huddinge University Hospital and is run in cooperation with the medical and neurological departments. There is a well-established and well-organized out-patient clinic where a doctor, nurse and a physical therapist follow the progress of the patient at regular intervals. The rehabilitation of stroke patients is carried out in general medical or neurological wards and continues on long-term care units or in other rehabilitation institutions.

One of the objectives for physical therapists in the project is to increase the quality of rehabilitation by running different educational programmes. To achieve consistency in methods of rehabilitation of stroke patients among paramedical professions, the physical therapist in the project established a forum. The aim of these regular meetings is the development of guidelines for technical equipment, treatment procedures, and education of nursing staff. The present report will focus on educational programmes for nurses, nursing assistants and aids, occupational and physical therapists and relatives of stroke patients.

INTRODUCTORY PROGRAMME FOR NURSING AIDS AND ASSISTANTS

The physical therapist must maintain continuity in her treatment and adhere to certain principles to reach the goal in the patient's rehabilitation plan. In order to achieve an optimal result it is necessary that all nursing staff work according to the same principles, with a specific goal for each patient in mind. For the stroke patient to be motivated in the physical therapy department to use the affected side as much as possible, and then to have ward staff encourage the opposite, must surely be very frustrating for the patient.

There is evidence that increased muscle activity and increased input from the sound side gives the affected side a poorer chance of recovery (Taub, 1980). Even so, it is relatively common for patients to be encouraged to use the trapeze for transfers in bed or to use a single-hand-driven wheel-chair for mobility. These examples show a lack of continuity in the therapeutic surroundings. It is vitally important that the nursing staff become aware of these therapeutic principles and therefore are more able to give the patients correct verbal feedback when performing transfer or other ADL activities. Correct feedback is also an important factor in increasing the patient's motivation (Belmont et al, 1969).

The educational department at Huddinge University Hospital organizes a two-week introductory course for newly employed nursing aides and assistants who are without prior formal training. A two hour lecture is held by the physical therapist in the stroke project. This aims to emphasize the importance of keeping compensatory activity on the sound side as low as possible.

The educational programme

A. Symptomatology and recovery from stroke

The lecture begins with a brief explanation of motor, sensory, and perceptual dysfunction in patients with stroke. The importance of early mobilization (Stein et al, 1971; Feigenson et al, 1977) in the facilitation of motor recovery is pointed out. Furthermore, the nursing staff are urged always to approach the patients from the affected side to reinforce the correct initial position for transfer activities, and to avoid symptoms such as unilateral neglect (Diller, 1977).

B. Positioning in bed during the acute stage of stroke

A slide demonstration of appropriate bed positioning to avoid an increase of spasticity in flexion synergy of the arm and in the extension synergy of the leg is used (Sterner & Widen-Holmqvist, 1976).

The participants practise with each other in order to assess various positions. They also try incorrect positioning: i.e. the head of the bed too high, forcing the patient to lie in a slouched position, or sidelying with the undermost shoulder in excessive retraction (Figs. 8.1a and 8.1b). They are taught to support the affected side with:

Supine
— Normal alignment of head and shoulders.
— A pillow placed under the head and neck, not under the shoulders.
— The arm supported by a pillow, in elevation in relation to the heart.
— The shoulder held forward in abduction and external rotation from behind with a small pillow.
— The shoulder protracted by holding one hand in the patient's axilla as the other gently eases the scapula forward. This technique, in particular, should be well practised (Fig. 8.2).
— The elbow placed in extension.
— The forearm and hand in supination.
— The hip supported from underneath to prevent external rotation and the knee supported with a folded towel to prevent hyperextension.

Sidelying on the sound side
— A pillow placed under the arm. The shoulder is well protracted and the elbow is held in extension. The hand is also supported.
— A big pillow supporting the back.
— A pillow supporting the affected leg with hip and knee maintained in flexion.

Sidelying on the affected side
— The affected shoulder well protracted and the elbow placed in extension.

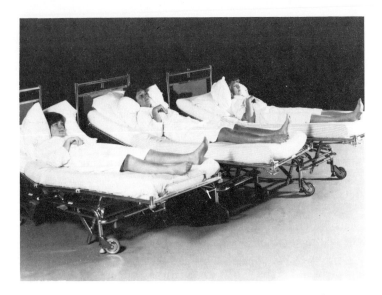

Fig. 8.1a

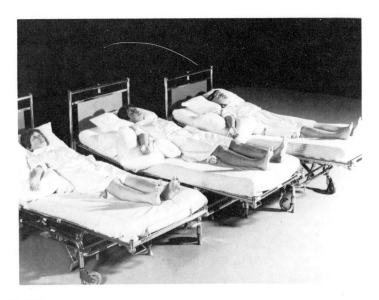

Fig. 8.1b

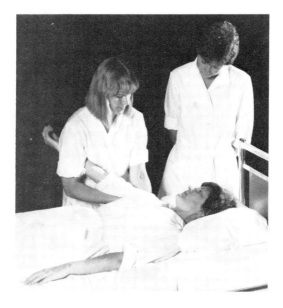

Fig. 8.2

— The leg flexed at the hip and knee. A pillow may be placed between the knees and/or behind the back.

C. Analysis of the sitting position

A slide demonstration on how a patient should sit to eat is used. The following components are emphasized:
— Both feet together on the floor.
— An even weight distribution.
— Flexed hips and extended trunk.
— Symmetrical trunk and the head held in midline.
— The affected arm supported on the table.
  The participants also assume various sitting positions and try drinking in an incorrect position so that they can appreciate the importance of the above mentioned components.

D. Analysis of standing up

The participants observe a person transferring from a sitting to standing position. The following components are emphasized:
— Feet together and pulled back for correct weight distribution.
— Flexion at the hips. The center of gravity is shifted forward.

— Raising to standing through extension of hips and knees.
— The weight evenly distributed on both legs in standing.
The participants try to realize for themselves how far forward the center of gravity actually has to get when standing up.

EDUCATION PROGRAMME FOR NURSING STAFF

The courses are run twice a year for nursing staff in ten different wards of the medical and neurological departments working with stroke patients. Each ward has 22 beds and about 7 nurses and nursing-aids.

The nurse in charge of each ward decides when to fit the course into the in-service educational programme. The course is divided into three one-hour sessions, during three consecutive weeks. The most suitable time during the day is when the morning and the afternoon shifts coincide. For the night shift the most suitable time is in the early evening.

It is of great importance that the nurse in charge encourages her staff to participate. Information regarding the course is also advertised on the notice board of the ward.

The physical therapist in the stroke project, in cooperation with the physical therapist in charge of the ward, runs the course. This cooperation facilitates the supervision of the participants during the practical sessions and makes association with the patients treated on the ward possible.

The course is held in the educational department of the hospital where both audio-visual equipment and beds are available. The three sessions are scheduled as follows.

Session one

A. Pathophysiology and symptomatology of stroke

Causes and risk factors of stroke are presented. The course of onset, recovery and prognosis is also discussed.

B. Motor dysfunction

The following aspects are described.
Immediately following the onset the affected side is in a paretic phase which can vary with time. After that, spasticity usually develops.

The spasticity develops in so called 'flexion' and 'extension' synergies. The flexion synergy is described as a shortening of the arm or leg and the extension synergy as a lengthening (Brunnstrom, 1970). Usually the flexion synergy dominates in the arm and the extension synergy in the leg.

With spasticity follows an inability to activate isolated muscle groups and a consequent difficulty in performing individual movements.

This involuntary, increased muscle tone can be increased by, for example, forced use of the intact side and by pain. Forced use of the intact arm occurs when the patient uses the trapeze for transfers in bed. The nursing staff are instructed to remove the trapeze as soon as the stroke patient is admitted to the ward. It is important that patients never become dependent on the trapeze for transfers. If they start to rely on it, it will take a longer time to learn to transfer in a normal way. Sometimes it is impossible to make the patient independent again.

C. Sensory dysfunction

The following aspects are described.

The patient may have a sensory dysfunction on his affected side and since he may not interpret touch, pressure, pain or temperature in a normal way, this side of the body is easily injuried. Sometimes the patient is not able to appreciate the position in which he has his arm and leg.

The participants are told to close their eyes and move one of their arms around and then to imitate this movement with the other arm. This exercise is used to make them aware of the importance of intact sensation for normal movement.

The following situations, in which stroke patients with sensory dysfunction can encounter problems, are pointed out to the nursing staff:

— The affected arm may hang down beside the wheel-chair without the patient knowing it, and be injured. The nursing staff are instructed to support the patient's affected arm on the wheel-chair table.
— Inability to perceive hot and cold.
— The likelihood of pressure sores: turning schedules should be used.

D. Perceptual dysfunction

The following aspects are described.

Perceptual dysfunction implies a difficulty in interpreting the information from our sensory organs; vision, hearing, sensation, smell and taste. This can result in disturbances of body image, body scheme, spatial relations and difficulty in recognizing and handling clothing and well-known objects, e.g. knife, fork, toothbrush and soap. The nursing staff's attention is focused on the importance of always approaching the patient from the affected side. This will stimulate the patient to turn his head to the affected side and look at this side of his body.

The nursing staff are instructed to place the bedside table on the affected side to further focus the patient's attention to this side. In this way it is easier for the medical staff, relatives and visitors to place themselves on the affected side of the patient.

If possible, the stroke patient's position in the room should be with his affected side to the entrance door. This makes it natural for the patient to turn to his affected side when someone enters the room.

E. Communication disorders

The following aspects are described.

Communication disorders can imply difficulty in understanding what is said, in finding the right word to say, or a combination of both. The patient may also have incoordination of the muscles used in speaking, which leads to incorrectly pronounced words.

The nursing staff are told to keep the following aspects in mind:
— Conversation and discussion in the presence of the patient should always include the patient.
— Staff should speak slowly. Short sentences with simple grammatic structures should be used, and the sentences formed in a way which makes it possible for the patient to answer without using complicated sentences. Staff should find out if the patient understands gestures better than verbal instructions.
— A close relative may be best suited to explain something to a patient with communication disorders.

F. Incontinence

The following aspects are described.

Incontinence of bladder and bowl may occur in the early stages, but usually disappears.

The nursing staff are urged to mobilize the patient as soon as possible so that he is able to sit on the toilet. Sitting and standing positions have a positive effect on bladder control. Furthermore, the nursing staff should pay extra attention to patients with communication disorders who may not be able to ask to go to the toilet.

G. Positioning in bed during the acute stage of stroke

The same slide demonstration on bed positioning, followed by the participants practising with each other, is used as that described in the 'Introductory programme for nursing aids and assistants' on page 187.

H. A manual with illustrations is handed out to each participant

The manual contains a summary of what is covered during the course. The participants are urged to read it and to be able to discuss the contents during the last session.

Session two

This consists of slide demonstrations (Sterner & Widen-Holmqvist, 1976).

A. Different pathogeneses of shoulder pain: treatment proposals

It is stressed that the humerus and scapula move together after the arm has been abducted above 20°. Furthermore, the importance of humeral external rotation in completing abduction greater than 120° is pointed out (Hoppenfelt, 1976). This is illustrated by slides, a skeletal model, and by the participants palpating scapular and gleno-humeral movement during arm abduction on each other.

In the stroke patient, the scapular-thoracic motion and the external rotation of the gleno-humeral joint may be restricted due to spasticity or decreased range of motion from other causes in the shoulder and trunk muscles on the affected side (Holmqvist & Kusoffsky, 1977).

If a patient's affected arm is forced into abduction without taking into consideration the scapular movement and the external rotation in the gleno-humeral joint, the structures around the shoulder may be traumatized. This can occur during routine patient care.

Shoulder pain in the stroke patient can often be caused by forced movements and trauma to the arm in ADL situations (Holmqvist & Kusoffsky, 1977). The following procedures should be used to prevent the development of shoulder pain:

— Correct placement of the arm and shoulder complex in resting positions as described above (introductory programme).
— Correct placement in the sitting position. A wheel-chair table should be used; when the patient sits in an ordinary chair the arm should be placed on a table.
— A 'sling' should not be used because it:
  (i) restricts motor recovery
  (ii) 'learned non-use' (Taub, 1980)
  (iii) keeps the arm in flexion synergy
  (iv) restricts the patient's ability to use normal balance reactions.

B. Body mechanics

The following aspects are emphasized.
The nurse should:
— Work close to the patient in transfer situations.
— Keep her back straight and be mobile in her legs.
— Transfer her body weight from one leg to the other instead of lifting or pulling with her arms.

C. Patient rolling from supine to sidelying

— The nurse should stand on the same side as the patient is turning towards and assisting him if necessary.
— The patient starts from the supine position with his hips and knees flexed. He lifts his bottom up and puts it down again in the opposite direction from which he wants to turn to. The trunk is then moved in the same direction.
— The patient holds his hands together and reaches with his arms towards the ceiling, while keeping his shoulders well protracted.
— Rotation and flexion of the neck to the desired side. Simultaneous movement of the arms to the same side.
— Rotation of the trunk. Patient rolls on to his side.

D. Sitting up from supine

— The patient should practise sitting up towards the affected side as this will further stimulate it.

— The patient rolls on to the affected side as described above.
— The patient moves his legs over the edge of the bed. He may need some assistance with his affected leg.
— The nurse should support the patient's head with one hand and the affected axilla with the other hand.
— The patient is instructed to sit up by lifting the head, laterally flexing the neck, and pushing against the bed with his arms.
— If necessary, in the sitting position, the nurse should assist the patient in keeping his head in normal alignment by asking him to look at her. She should stand directly in front of the patient. The following components are emphasized during retraining of sitting balance (Carr & Shepherd, 1982).
— Head in neutral position.
— Symmetrical shoulder position.
— Flexion of the hip and extension of the back.
— Body weight evenly distributed.
— Knees and feet together.

Session three

This also consists of slide demonstrations (Sterner & Widen-Holmqvist, 1976).

A. Standing up from a sitting position

— The patient starts in the sitting position with his feet on the floor.
— The nurse stands in front of the patient and supports his knees with her own.
— The patient holds on to her waist with his intact arm. The nurse assists him, if necessary, to do the same with his affected arm.
— She fixes the patient's forearms against her waist with her elbows.
— With her hands, she keeps a firm grip on the patient's upper arms.
— The patient is instructed to 'bend forward at the hips', keep his head up, and look at the nurse.
— The nurse bends her knees and keeps her back straight while following the patient's movement up to standing.
— The patient is instructed to shift his centre of gravity well forward, the body weight is first placed over his feet, and then the hips are extended.

— In the standing position the nurse holds on to the patient's hips to ensure an even distribution of body weight bilaterally.

B. Transfer to a chair or wheel-chair

— To focus the patient's attention on the affected side and to stimulate weight-bearing through the affected leg, the wheel-chair is placed on the patient's affected side parallel to the bed.
— The patient turns a quarter of the way around and sits down by flexing the knees while the body weight is kept well forward.
— The nurse follows the movement down to sitting while maintaining support and assistance to the patient's forearms and knees.

C. Eating

The following aspects are emphasized:
— Difficulty in chewing and swallowing, food expulsion, drooling, and lack of coordination between breathing and swallowing are examples of different eating problems (Carr & Shepherd, 1980).
— Factors which complicate the patient's performance are poor balance in sitting, difficulty in moving the head in relation to the body, decreased sensation, and abnormal reflex activity (Carr & Shepherd, 1982).
— Eating problems may be very frustrating to the patient and may affect his relationship with relatives and the nursing staff. It is important to pay attention to this problem at an early stage and improve the therapeutic surroundings during mealtime.

   Eating problems may lead to decreased food intake and malnutrition. The nursing staff are urged to consider the following aspects:
— The patient ought to sit, if possible, in an ordinary chair during the meal in the dining room on the ward. The wheel-chair should only be considered as a transportation tool.
— The transfer from wheel-chair to an ordinary chair is important psychologically. If, for some reason, it is impossible to move the patient to an ordinary chair, the following aspects should be considered by the nursing staff:
   (i) Remove the footrests and place the patient's feet on the floor.
   (ii) Move the wheel-chair close to the table.
   (iii) The armrests should be removed if they are not of the short type adapted for tables (desk arms).

(iv) If the patient has a wheel-chair table it should also be removed.
— Control the patient's sitting position as such:
(i) Feet together.
(ii) Flexion of the hips and extension of the trunk.
(iii) Body weight evenly distributed and forward in relation to the hips.
(iv) Both arms supported on the table in front of the patient.
(v) Head in neutral position and in some ventral flexion.
— If the patient needs assistance while eating the nursing staff should offer assistance from the affected side.
— Remind the patient to chew carefully and to keep the jaw and lips closed when not chewing.
The importance of a proper sitting position during meals is illustrated by the nursing staff practising the following:
— Attempting to drink in an incorrect sitting position, e.g. with the neck in dorsal extension and then in lateral flexion (Figs. 8.3a and 8.3b).

D. Wheel-chair and walker

The stroke patient should use a wheel-chair which is low enough to facilitate transfers and also permit reciprocal walking movements with the legs. A single-hand-driven wheel-chair is not to be used in order to avoid excessive input from the sound side. The nursing staff are also informed that the walker with handgrips should be used at first hand as a walking aid. This stimulates the use of the affected arm and encourages a more symmetrical postural alignment than does the use of a cane or a quadropod.

E. Reviewing the manual

Ten minutes are set aside for participants to ask questions and discuss the contents of the manual.

EDUCATIONAL PROGRAMME ON PERCEPTUAL DYSFUNCTION IN STROKE PATIENTS

Clinical experience indicates that stroke patients are often considered healthy if they have no motor deficit. However, the patient's ADL performance depends on both the level of motor function and on perceptual function (Bernspång, 1983). Perceptual

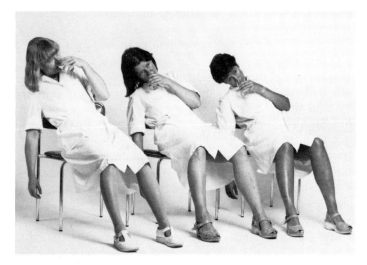

Fig. 8.3a

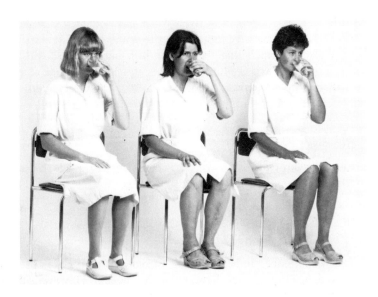

Fig. 8.3b

dysfunction is an important factor to be considered in the design of the patient's rehabilitation programme (Bernspång, 1983). Several examples have already been given of problems overlooked in the rehabilitation of stroke patients, for example: one patient refused to eat due to apraxia, another was not able to dial on the telephone due to acalculia, and a third patient could not use a pair of scissors due to agnosia. The list could easily be extended. The physical therapist, as well as other members of the stroke treatment team, must be aware of the possibility of perceptual disorders and treat them accordingly. So, our aim has been to increase the knowledge among all members of the treatment team from internal medicine, neurological and long-term care units regarding perceptual dysfunction in stroke patients and its influence on the rehabilitation process.

Screening test

A screening test on perceptual dysfunction with detailed instructions has been constructed in collaboration with the department of occupational therapy. The test can be used both by physical and occupational therapists and is designed for three different test situations: bedside, ADL and in the physical or occupational therapy departments. The aim has been that the screening test should be performed by the therapist as early as possible during the patient's hospital stay. In this way, recognition of perceptual dysfunction could be included early in the treatment programme. It is important that the nursing staff and relatives are informed of what consequences perceptual disorders have on the ADL performance.

At the bedside

At the bedside the following tests are carried out:
— Recognition of the relationship between different body parts.
— Perception of the paralysis.
— Right-left discrimination.
— Recognition of foreground from background.
— Performance of purposeful motor tasks on command or to imitate gestures.
— Understanding and recall of the position of different localities e.g. finding the way to the dining-room or the toilet on the ward.
— Judgement of depth and distance.

Activities of daily living

In ADL, perceptual problems often become more evident than at the bedside. The patient is observed dressing, eating and participating in hygiene activities. For example, the therapist focuses her attention on how well the patient handles different articles and parts of his clothing. Does the patient recognize the different parts and how does he plan his dressing? When the patient is eating, the therapist observes how well he is able to handle a knife, spoon and fork and how he drinks or sips through a straw.

In the therapy department

Here, a quiet room without distraction, when evaluating a patient's performance, is an advantage. The following tests are used:
— Drawing a man and a clock (to detect the presence of unilateral neglect).
— Copying a picture of a house and block constructions (to detect impairment in producing designs in two or three dimensions).
— Finger identification.
— Identifying three embedded pictures on a plate, figure-ground perception.
— Performing purposeful motor tasks in a logical manner with or without an object.
— Recognizing objects by handling, stereognosia.
— Reading a watch; handling money, the dial on a telephone; laying a tray; and preparing a letter ready to post.

The educational programme

The programme focuses on the following aspects:
a. Definition of perception.
b. Presence of perceptual dysfunction in patients with left and right hemisphere lesions.
c. Influence on ADL and the rehabilitation process.
d. Advantages and disadvantages in different treatment approaches; Sensory integration, transfer of training, compensation and adaptation (Siev & Freishtat, 1976)
e. Obstacles regarding validity, reliability and standardization of the screening test.
f. Factors complicating the patient's performance in test situations. Attention is focused on the following:

(i) When performing the screening test special attention must be paid to motor, sensory, visual, speech and language problems.

(ii) Perceptual dysfunction can be observed either in conjunction with the above mentioned problems or independently of them.

(iii) It must be remembered that sensory problems affect the evaluation of many perceptual problems: for example, it can bias the evaluation of unilateral neglect.

(iv) When receptive dysphasia is present it also influences the patient's performance.

(v) Visual field defects may cause symptoms similar to those caused by defects concerning spatial relations.

(vi) Motor problems interfere with the evaluation of apraxia.

g. Laboratory session in testing and treatment of distorted body image, spatial relationships, apraxias and agnosias.

The programme has been designed to suit different groups of the stroke rehabilitation team. Courses have been prepared for occupational and physical therapists together, while nurses, nursing assistants, aids and medical students have attended a more limited introductory programme.

Two videofilms have been produced in cooperation with the occupational and speech therapists, demonstrating how patients with perceptual dysfunction are tested. These films form a valuable part of the education programme.

Our experience is that the screening test is a helpful tool in identifying most patients with perceptual dysfunction. However, in patients with subtle disturbances the test may not be sensitive enough.

The education programme has resulted in an increased awareness and knowledge of perceptual dysfunction among the members of the stroke treatment team. It is our impression that it has both facilitated and deepened the nursing staff's and relatives' understanding of the stroke patient's problems.

INFORMATION PROGRAMME FOR RELATIVES OF STROKE PATIENTS

A cerebrovascular accident not only leads to a significant change in the patient's lifestyle but also affects, to a great extent, the relative's situation. Relatives often become anxious and frustrated, not knowing how to behave towards their ill relative who may have motor dysfunction, communication disorders, or a change in personality.

Brain-injured patients demand more personal contact and stimulating surroundings than other patients to be able to participate satisfactorily in a rehabilitation programme (Belmont et al, 1969). Members of the treatment team and relatives affect the patient's motivation with their support and positive influence. It is of utmost importance that the relatives feel confident in their new situation. This confidence is achieved when the relatives have no doubt that the patient is well taken care of. A relative who feels confident but who also has enough information about the disease is the person best suited to communicate with the patient. In this way relatives can also be of assistance to the staff in their work. So, it is of great importance that relatives obtain further information about the different dysfunctions of the stroke patient, and how they themselves can contribute to the long rehabilitation process after the hospital stay (Wells, 1974).

For this reason, relatives should meet as many members of the treatment team as possible during the hospital period. After the patient's discharge, contact with personnel at an out-patient clinic seems valuable. However, quite often a lack of continuity may threaten this desirable development. Published evaluation of group information for relatives of stroke patients indicates that it is an effective way to reduce worry and anxiety (Wells, 1974; Mykyta, 1976; Dza, 1978; Manuel, 1979). A series of group information sessions began at Huddinge University Hospital in 1981. A written invitation to participate in group information sessions was handed to relatives in conjunction with their visits to the ward or to the out-patient clinic. During the first trial period, group information was divided into three different sessions of one hour each, once a week.

The first session consisted of an introduction with a video film on stroke. This was followed by a talk from a doctor and a nurse about:
— Risk factors and causes of stroke.
— Examination procedures.
— Treatment and follow-up routines.

In the second session an occupational and a physical therapist spoke about:
— Different motor, sensory and perceptual dysfunctions.
— Transfers and ADL (Activities of Daily Living).
— Technical and orthopedic aids; home adaptation.

— How relatives can assist in stimulating and training the patient.

In the last session a social worker and a speech therapist discussed:

— Social consequences and resources.

— Speech and language disturbances.

The first trial period with group information consisted of 15 meetings and 34 visits by relatives. We thought that the number of relatives attending was too low in relation to the contributions of the members of the treatment team. Accordingly, we decided to try a new model.

During the second trial period the group information was decreased to one monthly session of one and a half hours. All members of the treatment team were represented. The second trial period resulted in four meetings with 25 visits by relatives. After every session the relatives were asked to fill in a questionnaire anonymously. The questionnaire consisted of 10 questions, and was translated and modified from Dzau (1978): see Table 8.1. We wanted to know whether relatives had increased their knowledge and whether this reduced worry. Furthermore, we wished to know whether contact with the treatment team had improved.

From data obtained through the questionnaire from the two first trial periods we came to the conclusion that two-thirds of the relatives felt better informed and less anxious. Three-quarters thought it was easier to put questions to members of the treatment team, while one-third was of the opinion that still more information was needed. In Table 8.1 the result of all questionnaires completed during 2 years are shown in per cent.

The attitude among the relatives was more positive during the first trial period, when the information was divided into three different sessions, than during the second: the probable reason being that the relatives were not able to avail themselves of all the information in one single session. However, we still did not feel satisfied with the way in which group information was organized in spite of positive replies from the questionnaire. Our impression was that relatives often had had difficulties in expressing their own problems. Experience from the trial periods has shown that it is important to begin each group information session with specific goals in mind instead of having standard information delivered in a monologue form.

At present, relatives are offered two group sessions where they are able to meet with two different representatives from the treatment team each time. The number of relatives is approximately ten

Table 8.1 Questionnaire administered to family members of stroke patients after attending the group information sessions. 64 questionnaires were completed altogether during two years.

Question	Responses %
1. Before attending the group information sessions I felt . . . . . because my relative has had a stroke:	
a. fearful and worried	66
b. slightly concerned	32
c. not worried and concerned	2
d. no answer	0
2. After attending the group information sessions I felt . . . . . about the stroke my relative has suffered:	
a. more worried	2
b. better and less worried	72
c. no change	23
d. no answer	3
3. Before the group information sessions I knew:	
a. almost everything about stroke	10
b. as much as I needed to know about stroke	28
c. incorrect information about stroke	3
d. nothing about a stroke	56
e. no answer	3
4. As a result of the group information sessions:	
a. I know more about stroke than I knew before	57
b. I learned nothing new	6
c. I learned as much as I needed to know about stroke	20
d. I still need more information	17
e. no answer	0
5. As a result of the group information sessions:	
a. I feel more comfortable visiting my relative	64
b. I feel the same about visiting my relative	34
c. I feel more uncomfortable visiting my relative	0
d. no answer	2
6. After the group information sessions:	
a. I understood the function of the rehabilitation team prior to the group information	9
b. I now know what the members of the rehabilitation team do for my relative	72
c. I still would like more information about the function of the rehabilitation team	17
d. no answer	2
7. After the group information sessions:	
a. it will be easier for me to ask questions of members of the rehabilitation team	78
b. it will not be any easier for me to ask questions of the rehabilitation team	0
c. I plan to ask questions as I did before the group information	17
d. no answer	5
8. After the group information sessions:	
a. I am still unclear about what the future holds for my relative	37
b. I have a good idea of what to expect from my relative from now on	56

Table 8.1 (cont'd)

Question	Responses %
c. no answer	7
9. Do you think that this way of presenting information is:	
a. suitable and clear	98
b. not clear	2
c. Preferred presentation is 0	
....	
10. Do you think that there is enough information?	
....	
Is anything missing?	
....	

To the last open question 70% indicated in different ways that they
thought the information was enough. 30% indicated that they
missed something. The list below are examples of what the relatives
commented on:
— better contact with the resident physician
— not enough time for questions
— more information from the social worker regarding different
   longterm care and rehabilitation possibilities
— more discussion with staff members about their own relative's
   situation.

each time. During the visiting hour the physical therapist contacts
the relatives on the ward, presents the group information, and
hands out a written invitation.

A few days before the group information session is scheduled,
relatives are reminded by a telephone call from the nurse at the
stroke out-patient clinic.

After a short introduction with information on the nature of
stroke, the relatives introduce themselves and discuss their own
specific problems. In this way the relatives guide the meeting.
Members of the treatment team have to adapt their presentation
according to the problems presented. An information pamphlet is
distributed to relatives for study at home. Information about
different patient associations is also given.

These group information sessions for relatives often lead to relatives accompanying the patient to the occupational, physical and
speech therapy departments which is of great value.

During the two years we have had group information sessions for
relatives of stroke patients, we have had the definite impression that
this contact is appreciated by the relatives. As is well known from
experience with other patient groups (Edhag et al, 1982), both
patients and relatives also benefit from contact with others who
have similar problems.

ACKNOWLEDGEMENT

We would like to thank Claes Helmers, Assistant Professor, Department of Medicine, Huddinge University Hospital, for his valuable help.

REFERENCES

Belmont I, Benjamin H, Ambrose J, Restuccia R D 1969 Effects of cerebral damage on motivation in rehabilitation. Archives of Physical Medicine 50: 507–11

Bernspång B 1983 Stroke rehabilitation: the influence of motor and perceptual dysfunction on ADL-performance. First European Conference Research in Rehabilitation, Edinburgh

Bobath B 1978 Adult hemiplegia: evaluation and treatment, 2nd edn. William Heinemann Medical Books, London

Brunnström S 1970 Movement therapy in hemiplegia. Harper & Row, Hagerstown

Carr J H, Shepherd R 1980 Physiotherapy in disorders of the brain. William Heinemann Medical Books, London, pp 333–334

Carr J H, Shepherd R B 1982 A motor relearning programme for stroke. William Heinemann Medical Books, London

Diller L, Weinberg J 1977 Hemi-inattention in rehabilitation: the evolution of a rational remediation program. In: Weinstein E A, Friedland R P (eds) Advances in neurology. Raven Press, New York, p 68

Dzau R E, Boehme A R 1978 Stroke rehabilitation: a family-team education program. Archives of Physical Medicine and Rehabilitation

Edhag O, Vourisalo D, Theorell T, Perski A, Bodin L, Kriegholm E, Rasch E 1982 Gruppinformation för hjärtinfarktpatienter möjlig väg minska antalet negativa psykiska effekter. Läkartidningen 79: 4280–4283

Feigenson J S, McDowell F H, Meese P, McCarthy M O, Greenberg S D 1977. Factors influencing outcome and length of stay in a stroke rehabilitation unit. Stroke 8: 651–656

Holmqvist L, Kusoffsky A 1977 Smärta i skuldran vid hemiplegi. Sjukgymnasten 5

Hoppenfeld S 1976 Physical examination of the spine and extremities. Appleton-Century-Crofts, New York

Manuel M 1979 Doing it the family way. Nursing Mirror June 21: 28–29, 34

Mykyta L J, Bowling J H, Nelson D A, Lloyd E J 1976 Caring for relatives of stroke patients. Age and Aging 5: 87–90

Siev E, Freishtat B 1976 Perceptual dysfunction in the adult stroke patient. A manual for Evaluation and treatment. Charles B. Slack Inc, New Jersey

Stern P H, McDowell F, Miller J M, Robinson R N 1971 Factors influencing stroke rehabilitation. Stroke 2: 213–218

Sterner E, Widen-Holmqvist L 1976 Functional positioning and transfers for a patient with hemiplegia. Sound slide program. Chartwell Bratt Ltd, Bickley, Bromley, Kent

Taub E 1980 Somatosensory deafferentation research with monkeys: implications for rehabilitation Medicine. In: Ince L P (ed) Behavioural psychology in rehabilitation medicine: clinical implication. Williams and Wilkins, Baltimore, pp 371–401

Wells R 1974 Family stroke Education. Stroke 5: 393–396

Annotated bibliography

Recognition of the scope of relevant literature is fundamental to understanding the change in approach which has occurred in the development of treatment and management of hemiplegia. A bibliography designed to give any awareness of the breadth of the background literature must therefore include not only the work of physiotherapists but that of others from many related disciplines. This bibliography makes no attempt to include all papers which mirror the current debates and uncertainties but concentrates on published material which condenses ideas and which has been found to be significant in the understanding of the problems posed by hemiplegia and of value in the development of treatment programmes.

Many of the texts focus on specific areas and include the work of specialists in a particular field. The texts listed also include many to which the contributors to this volume have referred, and which they have found valuable in formulating their ideas.

The bibliography is arranged in sections to assist further study but it must be recognised that for such a broad subject divisions are artificial and overlap will occur.

EPIDEMIOLOGY

Weddell Jean M, Beresford Shirley A 1979 Planning for stroke patients. Her Majesty's Stationary Office, London.
This study was designed to provide information for those planning the care of stroke patients in a defined population, and to describe characteristics of the total population and the stroke patients, the care available to those patients and its shortcomings. It is a comprehensive survey of the incidence of strokes in a community. A register was kept of all patients who suffered a stroke over a period of one year and the follow-up of this group extended to four years. It contains much detailed information including the social impact of stroke and the degree of support services available to patients. Recommendations are made for future areas of study. This book will be of interest to those wishing an overview of the problems posed by cerebrovascular disease and particularly for those planning long term services.

Weinfeld F (ed) 1981 The national survey of stroke. Supplement No. 1 to Stroke,
Vol 12. No. 2, pp I-1-I-91,
    Also available from:
    American Heart Association
    7320 Greenville Avenue
    Dallas, Tx 75231
    (Monography Number 75)
    or
    Dr Frederic Weinfeld
    Department of Health and Human Services
    Public Health Service
    National Institute of Health, NINCDS
    Office of Biometry and Field Studies
    Bldg. FED, Room 7C14
    Bethesda, MD 20205
This comprehensive epidemiological study was designed to provide statistics on
hospitalised stroke patients and provides a wealth of information. A stratified
probability sample design was used to obtain data representative of the entire
United States population. The sample consisted of 1846 acute stroke patients
hospitalised in 124 different acute general hospitals during 1971, 1973, 1975,
and 1976. The first two chapters of the report describe the need, purpose and
methodology of the study. The next four chapters report the clinical findings,
survival statistics and economic impact of stroke, and are the most interesting
for physical therapists and the most helpful for long-range planning of
comprehensive rehabilitation programs.

NEUROSCIENCES AND OTHER RELATED SCIENCES

Bach-y-Rita P 1980 Recovery of function: theoretical considerations for brain
injury rehabilitation. Hans Huber Publishers, Bern.
    The stated goal of this book is the provision of a scientific basis from which
therapeutic procedures for brain damaged patients may be developed. The
contributors, all with a firm grounding in basic science as well as a concern for
its clinical application, present experimental results which they consider have
particular importance in rehabilitation. Many aspects of brain plasticity are
discussed including major theories relating to recovery of function following
brain damage, and the influence of drugs on this recovery. All papers are likely
to be of interest to physiotherapists but that by Moore outstandingly so. From
a neuroanatomical view she proposes ten cardinal principles of (re)habilitation
which she acknowledges have been influenced by clinical experience and
common sense. Some of these will be immediately acceptable to
physiotherapists; others will perhaps prove more provocative.
    This book is to be commended to all who from a science base wish to
develop and refine their therapeutic programmes.

Feldman R G, Young R R, Koella W P (eds) 1980 Spasticity: disordered motor
control. Yearbook Medical Publications, Chicago.
    This is a collection of papers given at a symposium on spasticity and as well as
the full text of the papers it also includes the questions and discussion that
followed.
    The paper by Burke on the muscle spindle and the paper by Ashby et al on
vibratory inhibition of the monosynaptic reflex should be particularly useful to
physiotherapists as they present current concepts on the abnormality in spastic
man and therefore should help physiotherapists in their quest to determine
ways of correcting the abnormalities. It is only as the causes of spasticity
become clearer that treatment techniques can be developed and assessed.

Finger S, Stein D G 1982 Brain damage and recovery—research and clinical perspectives. Academic Press, New York.
In their preface the authors state that while planning this book they became intrigued by the whole question of recovery from brain damage and the relationship between observed recovery, underlying physiology, theory of localisation and beliefs about how the nervous system may function in health and disease.
    The authors discuss two important points. Firstly they identify the communication gap that exists between those who study recovery of function following brain damage, and those who might practically make use of new observations. Secondly they urge that those involved in this work are not constricted by current views and theories, but continue to explore and consider alternative views of brain function.
    The book has three clear sections. Firstly, a historical review considers the precursors to current ideas. The second considers recovery of function and neuroanatomical plasticity in a developmental perspective. Finally, the multitude of factors which may affect the outcome of brain injury and enhance or retard recovery of function are reviewed.
    The authors note that one of the most exciting things about current brain research is the opportunity for the development of many differing approaches and many new ways of thinking about how the nervous system works. Their excitement is contagious and for many physiotherapists this book will be both interesting and invigorating.

Gazzaniga M S, Ledux J E 1978 The integrated mind. Plenum Press, New York.
Mind and brain are often considered as separate areas of systematic study. It is not often that authors consider esoteric topics such as love and hate and attempt to provide a rational biological basis for these familiar phenomena. Utilising split brain studies, the authors of this book admirably attempt to associate brain mechanisms with the functions of the mind. The result is a compelling text which will provide readers with some biological postulations concerning such functionally vital areas as intelligence, language development, memory and conciousness. The book is eminently readable and presents material from an experimental mode. This book will be of considerable interest to physiotherapists who are interested in looking beyond the sensorimotor ramifications of brain damage.

Hecaen A M 1978 Human neuropsychology. John Wiley & Sons, New York
This is an excellent text for those wishing to gain a greater understanding of the higher order cortical dysfunctions seen in many stroke patients. The text contains chapters on aphasias, apraxias, disorders of visual and auditory perception (including agnosias), disorders of somethesis, somatognosis and memory. An excellent chapter on cerebral plaststicity and recovery of function is also included. The authors make extensive use of both animal and human research findings throughout their presentation.

Herman R M, Grillner S, Stein P S G, Stuart D G (eds) 1976 Neural control of locomotion. Plenum Press, New York.
This collection of papers was given at a symposium on the neural control of locomotion. The papers present recent findings regarding the control of locomotion in animals at all levels of the evolutionary tree including insects, fish, cats and man. A study of the evolutionary process regarding locomotion should help physiotherapists in an understanding of the neural control of locomotion in man, although it is important that findings in lower animals are not taken to be wholly applicable to man. However, the chapter by Pearson and Dysons shows the importance of hip position and limb loading in the initiation of stepping in cockroaches and cats. The chapter by Cook and

Cozzens suggests that the same parameters are important in the initiation of gait in man.

Illis L S, Sedwick E M, Glanville H J (eds) 1982 Rehabilitation of the neurological patient. Blackwell Scientific Publications, Oxford.
The stimulus for writing this textbook was the authors' perceived need for discussion on neurological rehabilitation which considered relevant basic sciences, rehabilitation principles and research findings. This text therefore explores rehabilitation possibilities for neurological patients and provides a forum for the exchange of relevant information and ideas.

Many recognised specialists have contributed to this volume which has three distinct sections. The first deals with the effect of change on the mature nervous system. In this the physiological response to damage is explored and consequent therapeutic implications discussed. Many interesting hypotheses are proposed. The second considers possible practical approaches to problems posed by damage to the nervous system. The final section explores novel approaches to neurological rehabilitation. Future possibilities which are based on research in engineering, the use of alternative sensory channels and repetitive stimulation of the nervous system offer exciting visions.

This book, particularly the first and third sections, has much to offer those actively involved in development of neurological rehabilitation.

Ince L P (ed) 1980 Behavioural psychology in rehabilitation medicine: clinical applications. Williams and Wilkins, Baltimore.
In the foreword to this book the Series Editor suggests that it contains 'sparks that can, and should, ignite an explosive revolution in rehabilitation'. The style of the book is one which will further achievement of such high aims by attempting to bridge the gap between laboratory study and clinical practice. Each chapter includes not only the work of leading scientists in the field of behavioural psychology but also discussion on possible practical implications. Many areas of rehabilitation are considered but the greater part of the book is devoted to areas which are of direct concern to physiotherapists treating the neurologically damaged patient.

The book is in three clear parts. The first considers the basic principles and methodology concerned and will be helpful to those less familiar with the theoretical background of the behavioural approach. The middle section on treatment and training is concerned with the use of behavioural techniques in the treatment of specific aspects of disability. It includes chapters on perceptual remediation programmes and feedback techniques for motor problems. The final section, entitled 'The experimental laboratory and beyond' presents basic research findings which will undoubtedly continue to influence physical therapy programmes.

This book contains much information which will be of value to those wishing to extend the behavioural psychology basis of their clinical practice.

Lance, J W, McLeod, J G 1981 A physiological approach to clinical neurology, 3rd edn. Butterworths, London.
In the preface to the first edition the authors comment that however brilliant the physiological advances made in the understanding of other species, they are profitless for man until applied to him. This text aims to bridge the gap between laboratory studies in neurophysiology and clinical neurological problems. The mechanism of various neurological symptoms and signs are, wherever possible, described in terms of disordered physiology. The authors throughout refer widely to recent animal and clinical research findings. Each section contains a clear summary of the main points and is fully supported by references which will enable further study to be made.

This book will be of value to those who wish to revise and extend their knowledge of current neurophysiology.

Luria A R 1975 The man with the shattered world, Penguin, London.
A personal account of disability from brain damage must have particular interest to those involved in this area of rehabilitation. This book is a remarkable account of the rehabilitation of a young soldier who had suffered an injury to the left parieto/occipital area of the brain. It consists of extracts from the patient's diary painfully recorded over many years, together with a compassionate and understanding commentary by a distinguished neurophsychologist. This is a disturbing glimpse of the world of the person with brain damage but allows some insight to this strange world.

Marteniuk R G 1976 Information processing in motor skills. Hold, Rinehart and Winston, New York.
The author describes this text as an attempt to present a basic overview of the processes underlying man's ability to perform and learn motor skills. A number of recent sources have argued that rehabilitation of a stroke patient is indeed an attempt to provide the opportunity for the patient to learn previously acquired skills which have been altered as a result of damage to the central nervous system. If these viewpoints have merit, this text will be most useful to physiotherapists wishing to obtain a thorough basic grounding in the theory of motor skills acquisition. The author describes performance from a human information processing viewpoint and this approach makes a pleasant departure from the neurophysiological models traditionally favoured by physiotherapists. As such, this approach is every bit as scholarly and probably has more relevance to physiotherapists than is presently realised. The processes described are known to apply to people with normal CNS function. It is reasonable to assume that they will also apply to people with brain damage, at least to some extent, although only applied research will answer this assumption.
This publication consists of four major sections. The first section introduces key concepts and defines terms, while the second considers the subject matter in more detail including perceptual mechanisms. The third section addresses learning of motor skills, and the final component applies the previous material and discusses the learning implications.

Payton O, Hirt S, Newton R 1977 Scientific bases for neurophysiologic approaches to therapeutic exercise: an anthology. F A Davis, Philadelphia.
This text is a collection of many of the original research articles that provide the basis for the neurophysiological approaches to therapeutic exercise. The text provides fascinating reading and a valuable historical perspective on the development of theory behind therapeutic exercise approaches. Of particular interest to therapists concerned with stroke are reports by Twitchell, Walsh, Simons, and Penfield. The anthology is a very convenient tool for those without access to extensive medical library collections.

Poritsky R 1984 Neuroanatomical pathways. W B Saunders, Toronto.
The author of this book claims that neuroanatomy is a study of wiring or circuitry. As such, this beautifully illustrated colouring book is designed to present neuroanatomy in a clear and concise format while also presenting some clinical correlates. The colouring function is designed to encourage the reader to engage actively in learning by highlighting the pathways being studied. The illustrations, which are clear and instructive, provide a useful three-dimensional perspective to the reader. This format, and the book in general, will be of particular interest for those who wish to review their neuroanatomy.

Roberts, T D M 1978 Neurophysiology of postural mechanisms, 2nd edn. Butterworths, London.
Those with a need for specialist knowledge of postural mechanism and control will find this comprehensive text useful. It is divided into four distinct parts which deal with the basics of posture, including basic neurophysiological concepts, the mechanics of posture, upright posture and the role of the nervous system. Although essentially a book for the specialist, many others will find the final section with its discussion on the interactive nature of the nervous system in the co-ordination of posture of considerable interest.

Rosenthal M, Griffith E, Bond M, Miller D 1983 Rehabilitation of the head injured adult. F A Davis Co, Philadelphia.
This text is included because many of the ideas presented in the book are applicable to stroke patients, particularly those related to motor assessment and motor retraining. The text highlights important research advances of the past decade, and provides a useful guide to clinical practice. Thirty well referenced chapters cover a wide variety of topics relevant to the management of the head-injured adult.

Walsh R N, Greenough W T 1976 Environments as therapy for brain dysfunction. Plenum Press, New York.
The content of this book examines the role of the sensory environment in brain dysfunction. The problem is addressed from the perspective of many disciplines ranging from basic neurobiology through ecology to developmental psychology. The book suggests that these sensory/environmental influences are strongly implicated as being of importance in treating brain dysfunction in its broadest terms. Much of the experimental evidence has been derived from animal models but the book addresses the appropriateness of generalizing this information to humans.
    This publication is of some importance clinically because of the emphasis placed by physiotherapists upon the sensory environment. Although the relevant research remains to be done, much of the content is consistent with present physiotherapy practice in the management of stroke. Consequently, physiotherapists practising in all aspects of the neurosciences will be interested in this work.

Williams M 1979 Brain damage—behaviour and the mind. John Wiley & Sons, Chichester.
This book considers the effect on different mental functions of disorders of the cerebral cortex. Each section begins with a description of clinical observation of disturbance, includes accounts of some underlying experimental investigation and proceeds to consider the basic anatomical background. Although written primarily for psychologists this book will be of interest to physiotherapists treating the outcome of brain damage. Of particular concern will be those chapters which consider disorders of perception, motor skills, bodily awareness and language.

Winter D A 1979 Biomechanics of human movement. John Wiley & Sons, New York.
In the words of the author, this book is designed as a resource for both the practitioner and researcher with its content applied to a spectrum ranging from the elite athlete to the physically handicapped. The areas of kinematics, kinetics, anthropometry, muscle and joint biomechanics and electromyography are covered with particular attention being paid to measurement and analysis techniques. Information is presented in an orderly fashion and each section concludes with a problem which utilises actual subject data. These problems are designed to test the reader's comprehension and reinforce understanding of

the material. There is a wealth of information in this text which is of relevance
to physiotherapists but it must be recognised that there is a great deal of
attention paid to technology and interpretation of data using sophisticated
mathematical techniques. This text therefore will be of most interest to
physiotherapists who seriously wish to study the biomechanics of human
movement and who are involved in research.

BIOFEEDBACK

Basmajian J V (ed) 1983 Biofeedback: principles and practice for clinicians, 2nd
edn. Williams & Wilkins Co, Baltimore.
This comprehensive textbook provides a foundation for both the theory and
practice of biofeedback. It contains contributions from thirty authors who
discuss in realistic terms the uses and limitations of biofeedback in a wide
range of therapeutic situations.

A review of essential neuroanatomy and neurophysiology forms an
introduction to the major sections of the book. In the first of these, Neurology
and rehabilitation, a complete chapter is devoted to stroke rehabilitation. This
deals with practical issues such as the selection of patients, feedback modalities
and the principles of biofeedback re-training. While emphasis is placed upon
total rehabilitation of the patient, specific problems such as subluxation of the
shoulder and foot-drop are clearly discussed. The control of spasticity is dealt
with in a separate chapter. This section also illustrates the value of biofeedback
in the re-education of patients following lesions of peripheral nerves, tendon
and nerve grafts, and in selected aspects of rehabilitation following spinal cord
damage.

Technical consideration reviewed in Part Five remind the reader of the basic
electronics involved and also discuss special devices which may be used either
alone, such as feedback goniometers, or in conjunction with computers. A
chapter on electrode placement will help to eliminate much trial and error
technique commonly found in this modality of treatment. A final section deals
briefly with biofeedback and research.

This book is highly recommended for both beginners and experienced users
of biofeedback. A comprehensive index permits easy referral to specific topics,
and the extensive reference lists included with each chapter enable readers to
pursue research interests in greater depth.

Grieve D W, Miller D, Mitchelson D, Paul J, Smith A J 1975 Techniques for the
analysis of human movement. Lepus Books, London
This small textbook deals with a range of modern techniques such as polarised
light goniometry, force plate analysis and electromyography, which are used in
the recording and evaluation of movement. The forty page section on
electromyography by D W Grieve covers the basic principles and gives a clear
and concise outline of the theoretical and practical considerations governing the
use of this technique.

Electromyography is defined as a very convenient and sensitive tool which
indicates when muscles are 'electrically alive'. It may therefore by regarded as
an indirect index by which the efferent activity of the nervous system may be
assessed. EMG equipment is discussed in relation to the characteristics essential
for accurate pick-up, recording and processing of the signal, and for data
collection and analysis. A discussion on the uses and limitations of surface
electrodes has particular relevance for the physiotherapist, restricted as she
normally is to the use of non-invasive techniques.

Special attention is given to the interpretation of the signal. Physical
properties of the motor unit and its contraction are discussed, factors which

will modify or distort the signal are identified, and the relationship between the electromyogram and mechanical parameters such as tension are explored.

The chapter ends with a short section on the value and versatility of computer analysis of the electromyogram. Various methods of processing the waveforms are described and their uses discussed. An extensive list of references is included for the reader desiring to pursue the topic in greater depth.

Schwartz G E, Beatty J (ed) 1977 Biofeedback—theory and research. Academic Press, New York.
Published in 1977, this book was one of the first to present the collective findings of a number of investigators engaged in biofeedback research. Its purpose as stated by the editors is, 'to provide a detailed, scholarly and comprehensive treatment of a larger series of recent experiments dealing with the learned control of central and autonomic functions.'

The greater part of the book is concerned with the use of biofeedback to monitor and control autonomic functions such as visceral motility and cardiovascular responses. Neuromuscular education is limited to the training of relaxation in stress and stress related disorders, and to the learned control of single motor units. While the latter demonstrates the degree of voluntary inhibition which may be applied to skeletal muscle by normal individuals, the book has nothing to say regarding stroke rehabilitation. Its value to the physiotherapist lies mainly in its portrayal of research principles as they apply to biofeedback therapy.

MOTOR LEARNING THEORY

Magill R A 1980 Motor learning: concepts and applications. Wm. C Brown Co, Dubeque, Iowa.
This book is designed to provide the undergraduate level student with the basic concepts related to motor learning. Content is presented as a series of concepts which are then applied to a variety of example situations and consolidated by means of a discussion which also examines the validity of the concept in the light of current research findings. The book is divided into three main sections referred to as units. These units introduce key concepts, examine factors affecting the learner and present theory related to the learning environment. This is a useful text for providing fundamental information and relating current theory to scientific method. A list of more specific reading is presented following consideration of each concept.

Sage G H 1977 Introduction to motor behaviour: a neuropsychological approach. Addison-Wesley, Reading, Massachusetts.
A neuropsychological approach has been used by this author in an attempt to bridge the gap between the physiology of the central nervous system and descriptions of human motor behaviour. A number of neuroanatomical and neurophysiological concepts are described followed by information, developed from research findings, concerning factors involved in motor skill acquisition and performance. A number of psychological concepts such as motivation and arousal are considered in the context of their effect on motor behaviour. An extensive bibliography is presented to permit further study of any component covered in this text.

Schmidt R A 1982 Motor control and learning: a behavioural emphasis. Human Kinetics, Champaign, Illinois.
Physical therapists are specifically named in the preface of this book as a group who may derive benefit from the content. Three sections consider introductory

concepts, motor behaviour and control, and motor learning and memory. The scientific method of quantifying theory is strongly emphasised and a number of figures.and tables clearly demonstrate the points being discussed. Current theory and associated research findings in the area of motor control are presented along with an extensive and most useful reference list. This book is suitable for those who wish to pursue the study of motor skills acquisition.

THERAPEUTIC APPROACHES AND METHODS

Benton L, Baker L, Bowman B, Waters R 1981 Functional electrical stimulation: a practical guide. Rancho Los Amigos Rehabilitation Engineering Center, 7601 East Imperial Highway, Downey CA 90242.
Rancho Los Amigos Hospital has been for years a leader in the development, application and research of methods for retraining motor function through the use of functional electrical stimulation techniques. In this practical guide the authors explain all the 'how-to's' of application, based on the extensive experience of the Centre. The manual contains many photographs and clear descriptions. Many techniques are applicable to rehabilitation of the stroke population.

Bobath B 1980 Adult hemiplegia: evaluation and treatment, 2nd edn. Heinemann, London
A bibliography concerned with treatment of adult hemiplegia would be incomplete without this text. It contains sections on evaluation, principles of treatment and techniques of treatment which enable physiotherapists to follow this therapeutic approach. Many of the concepts discussed, such as the importance of qualitative assessment of movement or the relationship between assessment and treatment, have provided the basis of further development in treatment programmes.
   The philosophy and methods described in this book have made a major contribution to the rehabilitation of the brain damaged patient.

Brunnstrom S 1970 Movement therapy in hemiplegia. Harper & Row, New York.
This classic text by the famous Swedish-American physical therapist should be part of every therapist's library. A theoretical framework and detailed practical guide to evaluation and treatment are provided. A useful method of describing motor recovery of different states is offered. The careful reader will probably be surprised at how similar many of the techniques advocated by Brunnstrom are to those developed independently by the Bobaths. The text also contains abstracts and citations of 25 original neurophysiological research articles relevant to the approach. This is quite helpful to those whose only language is English as many of these articles are published in German.

Carr J H, Shepherd R B 1982 A motor relearning programme for stroke. Heinemann, London
The development of this approach to relearning movement following hemplegia arose from the study of human movement, motor skill acquisition and theories of learning and motivation. The authors stress the importance of analysis of the patient's movement and subsequent identification of missing or abnormal components. Techniques for re-education of these components together with methods of progression are discussed.
   Common functional movements are used to exemplify this approach to rehabilitation. Each in turn is analysed and methods of retraining missing components are described in a fairly detailed manner. This section of the book is well illustrated by photographs which identify normal and abnormal movement patterns.
   Each chapter is supported by an extensive reference list enabling others to understand the development of the authors' approach.

Cotton E, Kinsman R 1983 Conductive education for adult hemiplegia. Churchill
Livingstone, Edinburgh.
Conductive education is described as being a new technique, developed in
Hungary, for rehabilitating partially paralysed adult patients. It differs from other
rehabilitation techniques in that the therapists' skill is relied upon less than the
patient's own active participation and initiative. The system is concerned with
teaching 'dysfunctional' persons to become functional by developing their
adaptive and learning abilities. Group work is the accepted format for this and is
the responsibility of the Conductor, whose task is the organisation and direction
of the timetable and day's routine, and the identification of appropriate functional
tasks. The book includes a brief description of the neuro-psychological and
educational background of the technique and a clear account of examples of
group tasks suitable for hemiplegic patients. This book will provide a useful
introduction to this approach to motor learning.

Farber S D 1982 Neurorehabilitation: a multisensory approach. W B Saunders
Company, Toronto
This text is designed to present a comprehensive approach to the management of
patients with disorders of the nervous system. The first chapter, which consumes
a substantial part of the book, considers functional neuroanatomy which is used as
the basis for the assessment and therapeutic procedures presented later. The
resultant multisensory approach presented by the author is based on the work of
Ayres, Bobath, Brunnstrom, Fay, Kabat, Knott, Rood, Voss and other
contributors by applying her own perspective, rationale and synthesisation to
these approaches. By describing and interpreting these approaches, this book
contributes to the relatively sparse literature in this area.
  Physiotherapists, working in the neurosciences, will find this book of interest
providing it is seen only as a theoretical perspective. To the generalist
physiotherapist, it is possible that the content of this book will only add to the
mystical confusion that already plagues this area of physiotherapy.

Siev E, Freistaf B 1976 Perceptual dysfunction in the adult stroke patient: a manual
for evaluation and treatment. Chas B Stack Inc., Thorofare, New Jersey
This book, designed originally for occupational therapists, will be of value to all
who are treating patients with perceptual dysfunction. The introductory chapter
describes, broadly, the deficits encountered, the approach to evaluation used by
the authors and the philosophy of the treatment they advocate. Subsequent
chapters deal with body image and scheme disorders, spatial relations syndromes,
apraxias and agnosias. Each chapter discusses common, and sometimes less
common, types of disorders encountered in clinical practice under three headings;
a description of the disorder, methods of evaluation and suggestions for
treatment.

Sullivan P, Markos, P, Minor M 1982 An integrated approach to therapeutic
exercise: theory and application. Reston Publishing Co., Reston, Virginia (a
Prentice-Hall Company)
The authors present a theoretical framework for developing an integrated
approach to the application of therapeutic exercise to all types of patients
(Chapters 1–7). Techniques from Proprioceptive Neuromuscular Facilitation
(PNF), Rood, Bobath and Brunnstrom approaches are blended, with an emphasis
on PNF and Rood techniques. Later chapters use clinical problems (e.g. Chapter
8, Hemiplegia) to demonstrate the application of the integrated approach.
Excellent photographs and detailed instructions for techniques are provided.

Wolf S L (ed) 1984 Toward excellence in physical therapy practice: exploring
clinical decision making processes. Davis F A, Philadelphia (16 contributors):
(may not be published until 1985—not yet in print).

This text documents the proceedings of the Conference on Comprehensive Clinical Decision-Making, held in Atlanta, Georgia, September 22–26, 1982.

The conference was designed as a follow-up to the 1966 Northwestern University Special Therapeutic Exercise Project (NUSTEP) conference. The main goal of the conference was to assist physical therapists in developing and improving clinical decision-making skills. The first several chapters analyse the theory and process of clinical decision-making. The remainder of the chapters, contributed by clinical specialists in physical therapy, use a case format to analyse the reasoning behind specific clinical decisions. Clinical problems from the areas of cardiopulmonary, neurology (including stroke), orthopaedics, pediatrics, and sports medicine are presented.

Index